UNIVERSITY OF NORTH CAROLINA AT CHAPEL HILL

DEPARTMENT OF ROMANCE LANGUAGES

NORTH CAROLINA STUDIES
IN THE ROMANCE LANGUAGES AND LITERATURES

Founder: URBAN TIGNER HOLMES

Editor: CAROL L. SHERMAN

Distributed by:

UNIVERSITY OF NORTH CAROLINA PRESS

CHAPEL HILL
North Carolina 27515-2288
U.S.A.

NORTH CAROLINA STUDIES IN THE
ROMANCE LANGUAGES AND LITERATURES
Number 262

'PUEBLOS ENFERMOS'

'*PUEBLOS ENFERMOS*':
THE DISCOURSE OF ILLNESS IN THE TURN-OF-THE-CENTURY SPANISH AND LATIN AMERICAN ESSAY

BY

MICHAEL ARONNA

CHAPEL HILL

NORTH CAROLINA STUDIES IN THE ROMANCE
LANGUAGES AND LITERATURES
U.N.C. DEPARTMENT OF ROMANCE LANGUAGES

1999

Library of Congress Cataloging-in-Publication Data

Aronna, Michael.
  "Pueblos enfermos": the discourse of illness in the turn-of-the-century Spanish and Latin American essay / by Michael Aronna.
  p. – cm. – (North Carolina Studies in the Romance Languages and Literatures; no. 262).
  Includes bibliographical references.
  ISBN 0-8078-9266-1
  1. National characteristics, Latin American. 2. National characteristics, Spanish. 3. Mental illness in literature. 4. Ganivet, Angel, 1865-1898. Idearium español. 5. Rodâ, Josâ Enrique, 1871-1917. Ariel. 6. Arguedas, Alcides, 1879-1946. Pueblo enfermo. 7. Spanish American essays – History and criticism. 8. Spanish essays – History and criticism. 9. Latin America – Moral conditions. 10. Spain – Moral conditions. I. Title. II. Series.

F1408.3 .A76   1999
909'.09756081 21 – dc21

99-042034

Cover art from Fructuoso Carpena, *Antropología Criminal* (1909). Madrid: F. Fé, p. 80 (SLG) by permission of the General Research Division, The New York Public Library, Astor, Lenox and Tilden Foundations

Cover design: Heidi Perov

ISBN 0-8078-9266-1

DEPÓSITO LEGAL: V. 4.190 - 1999

ARTES GRÁFICAS SOLER, S. L. - LA OLIVERETA, 28 - 46018 VALENCIA

TABLE OF CONTENTS

ACKNOWLEDGMENTS

Revised versions of some of the chapters of this book have appeared in the following publications: "Spain as Virgin" and "Seneca's Fig Leaf and the Medicalization of Sexuality" appeared in composite form under the title "Ángel Ganivet's *Idearium español*: Virginity, Fig Leafs and the Medicalization of History" in *Journal of Hispanic Studies* vol. 19, nos. 1, 2, 3 (December 1997); "The Pathology of Simulation in Public and Private Life" appeared under the title "The Vice of 'Simulation' and the Conflated Pathologies of Race and Moral Corruption in Alcides Arguedas' *Pueblo enfermo*" in *Imprevué*. 1, 2 (1997).

Through the years many people have contributed to this investigation through their teaching, their scholarship and their friendship. I am deeply indebted to the following professors and colleagues for their insights in the preparation of this study: Román de la Campa, Mario Césareo, Rosa Helena Chinchilla, Antonio Cornejo Polar, Edmond Cros, Jo Anne Engelbert, Bronwen Heuer, Victorien Lavou, Patrizia Lombardo, Sylvia Molloy, Adrián Montoro, Michelle Ortuño, Lisa Paravisini-Gebert, Julio Ramos, Michele Soriano, and Roger Zapata. Special thanks to Eva Bueno and to my teacher and friend John Beverley for reading and commenting upon initial drafts of the book.

Finally, I am most grateful to my partner Gail Freund who put up with me during the most anti-social moments of the "creative process" when any other sane person would have looked for greener pastures. I dedicate this book to her.

INTRODUCTION: THE DISCOURSE OF DEGENERATION AND ITS DISSEMINATION IN THE SPANISH AND LATIN AMERICAN NATIONAL ESSAY

The historical period generally referred to in European cultural and historical studies as "turn-of-the-century," roughly the years between 1890-1918, has for a long time been associated with a sensibility of collective cultural fatigue or exhaustion. This sensibility, commonly denominated by the generic, all-inclusive term "decadence," manifested itself in expressions of censure, frustration, impotence and, in some instances, blissful indifference regarding the accelerating pace of the social, cultural and economic transformations realized by the entry of the logic and structure of industrial capitalism into all levels of life. The social discipline inaugurated by this transformation permeated the private and public spheres, rigidifying and antagonizing relations between the sexes, social classes and ethnic groups.

This social transformation was scientifically sanctioned by the biological doctrine of evolution in a discursive leap which projected the theories and beliefs of natural history on to human social, cultural and economic history. Within this mixing of evolutionary, economic and political discourses, the social antagonisms engendered by this allegedly "evolutionary" social transformation were simultaneously constructed as the processes of economic competition and natural selection. At the intra-national level, the benefactor of this organicist theorization of socio-economic antagonism and exploitation was the male, European bourgeoisie whose dominance over women, peasants, workers and ethnic minorities was simultaneously constructed as a biological, moral and rational manifestation of superiority. At the international level the evolutionary doctrine of the "survival of the fittest" provided renewed scientific and moral legitimacy for imperialism throughout Africa, Asia, and Latin America.

Yet the regional unevenness of this transformation, its intrinsic inequality and the social resistance it provoked, within the hegemonic European powers as well as their colonies, undermined one of the basic conceptual premises of this concept of evolution, namely, the Enlightenment belief in *man* as an inherently rational being. If this belief in man's innate rationality was true, late nineteenth century bourgeois society was faced with an ideological contradiction summarized in the following questions: why was this process of economic transformation, national state consolidation and transnational exploitation so conflictive?; why the continuation of poverty and misery within the wealthy states of Europe?; why the civil, international and imperialist wars of the late nineteenth and early twentieth centuries?; why was Europe justified in the subjugation and exploitation of colonial non-white peoples? The resolution to this contradiction, the European (and North American) intelligentsia reasoned, was that not all of humankind was rational and thus capable of evolutionary progress.

As Enrique Dussel has demonstrated, the intellectual basis for the exclusion of the vast majority of the world from the material benefits of reason and modernity was already present within the concept of Enlightenment. This exclusionary clause was provided by one of the principal articulators of Enlightenment thought, the German philosopher Immanuel Kant. Kant premised the development of reason, and thus of modernity, on an anthropomorphic, teleological process of "maturation" from an inherently sinful state of youthful sloth and irrationality, to an adult state of discipline and reason. As Dussel affirms, the effort invested to bring about this "evolution" towards rationality implies a moral superiority for the "enlightened" and a concomitant immorality for the "irrational": "For Kant, immaturity or adolescence are culpable states, laziness and cowardice their ethos: the *unmundig*" (68). In this way, a hegemonic, European modernity was personified in the terminology of morality and maturation, while a subaltern European (Spain, Italy, Eastern Europe) and African, Asian and Latin American premodernity was associated with immorality and childhood.

This intricate relationship between reason, modernity, national development and maturation was enhanced by Hegel. Hegel stated that Africa, Asia and the Americas were "immature" inasmuch as they were ontologically situated in the state of nature, namely, a state which is opposed to consciousness. For Hegel, nature, and the non-Europeans who live in a perpetual state of nature, remain in an ahistorical, preconscious state of being incapable of maturation or evolution. The social, cultural and political manifestations of these naturally "immature" peoples are judged by Hegel to be incommensurate with the progress of the universal spirit, and as such, are found to be accidental or inconsequential to history. Here we have two key recurring themes: 1) that nature is immature, imperfect, and corrupt; 2) that nature is outside of consciousness and history; it exists as Other in relation to the Idea.[1]

This anthropomorphic, developmental model of modernity and reason called for a system of knowledge capable of articulating the differences between these stages of mental growth. Accordingly, as Carl Schorske points out, the model of "rational man" was discarded in favor of another model capable of explaining this biologically justified inequality: "Traditional liberal culture had centered upon rational man, whose scientific domination of nature and whose moral control of himself were expected to create the good society. In our century, rational man has had to give place to that richer but more dangerous and mercurial creature, psychological man" (4).

The construction of psychological man enabled society to explain its social inequality and conflict not in terms of poverty, uneven development or the unequal distribution of wealth and power, but rather as pathology it thus authorized psychologists and their allied sexologists, criminologists and ethnologists to define the marginality of specific social, cultural and ethnic sectors as the manifestation of these groups' inherent irrationality, a condition rooted in abnormality or sickness. As Michel Foucault indicates, (in the following passage from *The Birth of the Clinic*,) it was not merely the content of biological and psychological theory that facilitated the medicalization of socially marginalized groups, but rather it was the structurally and functionally bipolar nature of this theory's articulation which made this classification possible:

> Furthermore, the prestige of the sciences of life in the nineteenth century, their role as model, especially in the human sciences, is

---

[1] Hegel, *Philosophy of Nature*: "Nature has presented itself as the Idea in the form of *otherness*. Since therefore the Idea is the negative of itself, or is *external to itself*, Nature is not merely external in relation to this idea (and to its subjective existence Spirit); the truth is rather that *externality* constitutes the specific character in which Nature, as Nature, exists" (sic).

> linked originally not with the comprehensive, transferable char-
> acter of biological concepts, but, rather, with the fact that these
> concepts were arranged in a space whose profound structure re-
> sponded to the healthy/morbid opposition. When one spoke of
> the life of groups and societies, of the life of the race, or even of
> the 'psychological life,' one did not think first of the internal
> structure of *the organized being*, but of the *medical bipolarity of
> the normal and the pathological.* (35)

In this way the medical and psychological disciplines discarded
the model of "health" for a prescribed model of "normality" based
on abstract, purely theoretical standards. "Sickness" was redefined
as the inability to meet these standards. Social organicists readily
applied this concept to society. Crusading, civic-minded psychologists, medical doctors, public health officials and criminologists
medicalized the working class, the *lumpen proletariat*, criminals,
ethnic minorities, "revolutionaries," prostitutes and women in general as "abnormal" or "sick." In this way those elements of society
who questioned the inequity of the system, either through the mere
fact of their poverty, through social protest and sexual or criminal
"deviancy" were medically marginalized. Moreover, the shift from
medical to social discourse was in itself a logical consequence of the
consolidation of the former. For as Foucault indicates, the very process of the professionalization and standardization of medicine was
linked to the state in its administrative and policing functions.[2]

In a larger context, the medicalization of the subaltern was a
fundamental task of modernity. The drive to isolate and classify the
organically and socially ill was part of a greater project to rationalize, modernize and industrialize the nation. Fulfilling this need, the
function of the discourse of degeneration was to determine which
groups and practices constituted biological and cultural obstacles
to modernity, to diagnose the illnesses afflicting these groups and to
develop treatments or solutions.

---

[2] In *The Birth of the Clinic*, while referring to a late 18th century document,
Foucault gives an account of the social and political authorization of medicine:
"And yet, in the final analysis, when it is a question of these tertiary figures that
must distribute the disease, medical expertise and the doctor's supervision of social
structures, the pathology of epidemics and that of the species are confronted by the
same requirement: the definition of a political status for medicine and the constitution, at state level, of a medical consciousness whose constant task would be to provide information, supervision, and constraint, all of which 'relate as much to the po-
lice as to the field of medicine proper'" (26).

In the advanced centers of Europe, the national mission of degeneration theory was realized throughout the discursive field. Philosophers, historiographers, psychologists, biologists, physicians and novelists of varying political ideologies such as Bagehot, Bourget, Carlyle, Clarín, Darwin, Fouillée, Gobineau, Guyau, Hegel, Janet, Le Bon, Lombroso, Macaulay, Morel, Nietzsche, Nordau, Ribot, Ruskin, Schopenhauer, Spencer, Taine, Tolstoy, Weininger and Zola endeavored to determine the physiological and psychological roots of the nation's marginal constituencies.

In the context of nineteenth-century thought, the disciplinary boundaries between the idealist philosophical discourses of degeneracy and the specifically psychological, phrenological and clinical discourses of the same were not fixed. This becomes particularly evident if one examines the role of the German philosophers Kant, Hegel, Schopenhauer and Nietzsche in the discourse of national illness.

As indicated earlier, both Kant and Hegel were central to nineteenth-century discourses concerning progress, modernity and the nation. Their attractiveness lay in their claim to systematic, scientific and mathematic rigor. It is precisely for this reason that their pessimistic and unfounded conclusions concerning Spain and the Americas call into question the legitimacy of their method.

Kant based his assumptions on the Americas on a mixed-brew of documentation and personal caprice. As did Hegel after him, Kant rather uncritically accepted the accounts of travelers who recorded their impressions of the Americas and the Americans. Inasmuch as these travelers were more often than not missionaries and other officials of empire, their accounts were informed both by their vocational investment and their pre-conceived European fantasies concerning the New World. On the scientific side, Kant borrowed from celebrated eighteenth-century naturalists who were notorious even then for their slanderous views concerning the health of the plant, animal and human life-forms of the Americas such as Buffon and de Pauw. As Antonello Gerbi has demonstrated, these two naturalists extrapolated a polarized system of comparative botany, zoology and "anthropology" from the accounts of colonial travelers. The resulting theories of Buffon and de Pauw range from a crude climatic-topographical determinism to ludicrously fantastic claims about the frailty or degeneracy of American flora and fauna. Both Buffon and de Pauw repeat colonial accounts of cowardly lions, mute birds, frigid natives and lactating males with the "objective" authority of science.

Armed with this kind of scientific documentation, Kant articulated a theory of the sublime which excluded women, Asians, Africans and the indigenous peoples of Central and South America. In his *Observations on the Feeling of the Beautiful and Sublime*, Kant departs from differences in gender in order to establish a hierarchy of national character. In short, Kant argues that women and, to varying degrees, all non-white peoples, are limited to a sphere of sensory experience at best. As a consequence, Kant asserts, women, the majority of caucasian men, and all non-whites lack the capacity for rational meditation. In the absence of reason, this overwhelming majority is incapable of exercising the freedom to choose virtue. For Kant, all of humankind, but for a select minority of elite caucasian men, possesses at best an aesthetic virtue which coincides with their taste or sensual nature. In this sense, women and nonwhites share a physical propensity for immorality, a theme which is frequently repeated in the literature of degeneration. Moreover, as Nancy Ochoa has affirmed, by equating the lack of virtue with an aesthetic, or in Kant's terms, a "beautiful understanding," Kant undermines what he characterizes as the feeling of beauty and dignity inspired by the beautiful (25). Thus a seed of moral doubt is lodged in aesthetic contemplation, a dilemma which is, as we shall see later, a recurring preoccupation in *Ariel*, a text written by the Uruguayan José Enrique Rodó.

Specifically with regard to the Spanish national character, Kant, the voice of progress and capital, negatively associates the Spaniard with the backwardness of Africa, the Middle Ages and the "sublime" brutality of the Black Legend, as in this passage from his *Observations*: "In his composition little of the kind and gentle benevolence is to be encountered; thus he is often harsh and indeed quite cruel" (100). As we will see, this notion of innate Spanish cruelty and arrogance has become a tenet of the doctrine of Spanish, and through extension, Latin American mestizo inferiority.

Writing nearly a half-century later, Hegel compounded the scientific error of Kant concerning the Spanish and Latin American character. In *Lectures on the Philosophy of World History*, Hegel's reliance on seventeenth-century accounts of colonial missionaries calls into question the systematic integrity of his claims. Likewise, Hegel's reiteration of the by then repudiated naturalism of Buffon and de Pauw further undermines the rigor and modernity of his argument.[3] More in keeping with contemporary science was Hegel's belief in elements of climatological and telluric determinism, two potent tools of nineteenth-century degeneracy theory.

Also following Kant, Hegel promulgated the Black Legend. He described the Conquest as an avaricious and cruel enterprise fueled by the "dregs" of Europe and a Catholic mentality. In the classic rhetoric of degeneracy theory, Hegel relates how the Spaniards, displaced in the tropics of the Americas, reverted to their worst propensities and transmitted their faults to the Creoles and mestizos. In this way Hegel reinforced the linkage between alleged Spanish and Latin American inferiority.

Hegel's considerable significance in the polemic concerning Latin America's alleged degeneracy is undoubtedly linked to his systematic consolidation of the time-worn notion of Latin America's geological, and more importantly, physical youth. The idea that the indigenous peoples of the Americas lived in a state of childlike innocence and ignorance is one of the foundational myths of the literature of "discovery" and colonization. Yet Hegel modernized this notion by incorporating it into his universal theory for understanding world history. Of great importance to our consideration of the discourse of national illness is the slippage in Hegel's thought between the categories of immaturity and impotence. In the *Lectures* he speaks of the indigenous Americans as "unenlightened children" who are physically unable to provide labor. According to Hegel, this physical impotence of the indigenous Americans necessitated the African slave trade.

Yet this negative view of youth is contradicted in his appraisal of classical Greece as the youthful, adolescent phase of world history. Here the category of youth is brimming with physical vitality and spiritual promise. Unlike the characterological immaturity impugned to the Americas, this state of adolescence is a vulnerable, transitory state capable of being properly or improperly cultivated. For, as Hegel affirms, the vital, sensual aesthetic of ancient Greece was morally unsound, an anxiety we will have occasion to examine at length.

---

[3] As Gerbi has demonstrated, the nineteenth-century Prussian naturalist Humboldt passionately refuted the notion of Latin America's zoological and botanical inferiority (417).

This theoretical confusion over the pathological or developmental nature of youth greatly concerned Latin American thinkers who promulgated or repudiated the notion of national illness at the end of the nineteenth century. As we will see in our consideration of Rodó's *Ariel* and the Bolivian Alcides Arguedas' *Pueblo enfermo*, the conflicting yet coexisting notions of degenerate and rejuvenating youth are inescapably linked regardless of their optimistic or pessimistic appropriations.

Schopenhauer and Nietzsche are important to our consideration of the discourse of national illness in Spain and Latin America not so much for what they said about a Latin or Hispanic character, but rather for their articulation of the linkage between volition, instinct, desire and restraint in the perception of turn-of-the-century "soul sickness." Not only did these two philosophers conceptualize this perceived cultural malaise, rather they lived it. In this sense these philosophers share a greater spiritual and existential affinity with the Spanish and Latin American authors of this discourse. Their concentration on pathologies of the will arising from both somatic and spiritual imbalances places them at the table with contemporary psychologists, sexologists and phrenologists who diagnosed neurological-sexual disturbances at the individual and social level.

In *On the Will in Nature*, a text in which Schopenhauer defends his intellectual property from plagiarism by phrenologists and physicians, Schopenhauer reasserts the primacy of the "unconscious will" as the source of health and disease. Inasmuch as the will has primacy over the body for Schopenhauer, its stimulation or lack thereof can account for states of health or disease. Just as health must be mediated through the will, illness is tied to its frustration. Schopenhauer's characterization of the will as the drive to procreate openly asserts that which, as we shall see later, authors like the Spaniard Ganivet and the Uruguayan Rodó seek to repress, namely the conflicted sexual nature of their anxiety or "soul sickness." It is in this light that I interpret the following passage from Schopenhauer's *The World as Will and Representation* as a precursor of aboulia, that psychological illness characterized by a lack of both volition and desire which, as we shall see, recurs throughout Spanish and Latin American treatises on degeneration:

> Now the nature of man consists in the fact that his will strives, is
> satisfied, and strives anew, and so on and on; in fact his happi-

ness and well-being consist only in the transition from desire to
satisfaction, and from this to a fresh desire, such transition going
forward rapidly. For the non-appearance of satisfaction is suffering; the empty longing for a new desire is languor, boredom. (1:
260)

Yet despite this apparent embrace of the will and its libidinal
nature, Schopenhauer promoted the idea of chastity as a means of
strengthening the intellect and promoting self-knowledge at the expense of the will. This contradictory notion is a particularly important juncture in the discourse of degeneration. For many theoreticians of spiritual and corporal enervation of the late nineteenth-
century, degeneration was synonymous with the fatigue of man's
vital functions. Given the perceived connection between the will
and sexuality, this "spiritual exhaustion" was associated with illicit
or excessive sexual activity. Subsequently, there was an obsession
with the retention of what was euphemistically known as "vital internal energy." Thus, to enliven the spirit, sharpen the intellect and
heal the body, physicians and national diagnosticians often prescribed a program of individual or social abstinence.

Nietzsche, one of the most provocative exponents and critics of
the discourse of degeneration, signaled the paradoxical nature of
this position. In his essay, "What is the Meaning of Ascetic Ideals?," Nietzsche affirms that denying the will is an act of self-depri-
vation that enervates both mind and body. Moreover, Nietzsche asserts, using Schopenhauer's terminology to ridicule the latter, that
asceticism further objectifies the sexual organs, making the disinterested contemplation of the beautiful impossible. Thus, Nietzsche
concludes, chaste aesthetic meditation is not a means for self-healing,
but rather constitutes a displaced mode of self-arousal and gratification. In this way Nietzsche derided the sanctimonious medical
tone of the soothsayers of cultural degeneration as in the following
passage: "But is he really a *physician*, this ascetic priest? We have
seen why it is hardly permissible to call him a physician, however
much he enjoys feeling like a 'savior' and letting himself be revered
as a 'savior'" (*Genealogy* 129).

This is the theoretical impasse of self-diagnosis and healing that
made Nietzsche such a central figure in turn-of-the-century Spanish
degeneracy theory. Nietzsche anticipates the Generation of '98's
dilemma of international withdrawal and self-contemplation, an op-

eration which was understood in terms of revitalizing the national will and spirit. The theoretical confusion concerning the concomitantly desired healing of the will and improved self-knowledge put into play conflicting notions of pathologies of the will and disinterested meditation as discussed earlier.

In Latin America, the idea that the nations and cultures of Latin America were youthful intensified this concern. Immaturity invoked notions of vulnerability and precocious corruption. If cultural regeneration rested on the proper guidance of the youth of Latin America, then the model for such guidance was of crucial importance. Here Nietzsche expresses similar concerns. Like many Latin American thinkers of his day, Nietzsche repudiated what he perceived as the utilitarian and philistine culture of nineteenth-century capitalism and democracy. As did the national intelligentsia throughout Europe and Latin America of his day, he sought refuge from the present in an idealized and eternally "youthful" Hellenic tradition fraught with its own contradictions on which he imposed his own conditions. Likewise, Nietzsche's tumultuous relation to the music of Wagner approximates the troublesome relation between Latin American theorists of degeneration and the decadent literature of such authors as Huysmans, Bourget and Wilde. Nietzsche's fascination with Wagner and his subsequent denunciation of the latter as a corrupter of youth mirrors the Latin American reaction to the turn-of-the century literature of decadence. [4]

Throughout Europe and Latin America, turn-of-the-century theoreticians of degeneracy held the attention of the state, and, in some instances, occupied governmental posts. The influence of their thought was enacted in governmental policy initiating changes in the penal code, the sanitary and hygienic standards of private and public space, the regulation of prostitution, the reform or establishment of public education, the military, the treatment and confinement of the ill and the insane, the persecution of and discrimination against allegedly inferior ethnic minorities such as Jews and Gypsies.

---

[4] In the *Case of Wagner* Nietzsche declares: "One pays heavily for being one of Wagner's disciples. I observe those youths who have been exposed to his infection for a long time. The first, relatively innocent effect is the corruption of taste. Wagner has the same effect as continual consumption of alcohol: blunting, and obstructing the stomach with phlegm" (184).

If the discourse of degeneration fulfilled a key role in the rationalization of uneven and unequal development in the advanced centers of liberal democracy, capitalism and industrial modernization, its significance in the vastly underdeveloped regions of peripheral Europe and Latin America was far greater. At the close of the nineteenth century in nations such as Spain and in those of Latin America, the systemic modernization characteristic of the advanced metropolitan centers of Europe had hardly begun. Much to the consternation of the Spanish and Latin American intelligentsia, the progress attributed to the allied forces of industrialization and parliamentary democracy under capitalism was conspicuously absent from their own nations. Reproducing the critical blind-spot of European social organicists regarding the socio-economic and political necessity of underdevelopment for the modernized hegemonic center, many Spanish and Latin American intellectuals examined their own populations in search of internal psychological, racial, criminal, moral and sexual deficiencies which would explain their own regions' or nations' weak and exaggeratedly uneven entrance into modernity. The result of this introspection was a series of essays in both Spain and Latin America which accounted for underdevelopment through psychological and medical explanations which found their nations to be too sick, immature, un-evolved and "feminine" to possess the rational and moral qualities necessary for national progress.

As Sylvia Molloy has stated, the Latin American appropriation of the discourse of European degeneration can be viewed as a discursive attempt to achieve, or rhetorically conjure, the modernity so desired by the Latin American intelligentsia. In this sense, authors such as Martí, Darío, and Rodó in Latin America did not wish to confirm the racial condemnation inherent in the discourse of degeneration, but rather sought to extract its promise of evolutionary regeneration, or as Molloy eloquently states: "Paradoxically then, the appropriation of European decadence by Latin America was less a sign of degeneration than an occasion for regeneration: not the end of a period but an entrance into modernity, the formulation of a strong culture and of a new historical subject" (191). Yet as Molloy suggests, just which regional, ethnic and class cultures and subjects would accompany Latin America into modernity would be determined by the pessimistic side of degeneration theory in Latin America.

In this context it is important to remember that the theories of degeneration constituted much more than a discursive accompaniment of modernity. The discourse of degeneration in Latin America, as in Europe, was actualized throughout social, political and cultural institutions. In an attempt to stimulate modernization, the discourse of degeneration brought about "reforms" in education, the courts, the political system, medicine and psychiatry and provided a scientific basis for the rationalization of the curtailing of civil rights and the persecution of racially, sexually and socially subaltern groups through direct repression and discriminatory legislation.

The social enactment of the discourse of degeneration in Latin America was facilitated by the lack of differentiation between cultural and political intellectuals. This continuity between cultural and political discourse and its protagonists was itself the product of economic underdevelopment which was also manifested in the underdevelopment and non-professionalization of the disciplines of knowledge. In the absence of an institutional, disciplinary division of knowledge, literature, philosophy and science commingled to fill the void created by the lack of a developed field of social sciences. A contemporary participant in this process, the Nicaraguan poet Rubén Darío, characterized the confluence of medicine and literature in an article on pathological criticism: "En tanto que la literatura investiga y se deja arrastrar por el impulso científico, la medicina penetra al reino de las letras; se escriben libros de clínica tan amenos que una novela" (453). In Darío and others like him we witness two phenomena characteristic of late nineteenth century and early twentieth century intellectual production in Latin America: the Latin American man-of-letters who writes literary, anthropological and sociological texts, like the novelist-sociologist-historiographer Alcides Arguedas; the development of a body of literature which does not draw exclusive distinctions between fiction, historiography and natural history, a tradition that had been promoted by Andrés Bello in his *Autonomía cultural de América Latina* of 1848 or Sarmiento's *Facundo*. This epistemological continuity was heightened by the fact that the essayists discussed in this study, Ganivet in Spain and Rodó and Arguedas in Latin America, occupied official posts within government and public education.

Although we will delineate two distinct socio-historic and intellectual trajectories for the discourse of national illness in Spain and Latin America, an argument can also be made for the commonality of their diagnosis. Due in part to their colonial or semi-colonial relationship and resulting underdevelopment (for Latin America at the hands of Spain and then England and for Spain at the hands of European finance capital and its own intransigent, aristocratic and ecclesiastical classes), Spain and Latin America encountered modernity carrying similar cultural, economic, political and ideological baggage. John Beverley has elaborated on these interrelated structures of dependency and underdevelopment in Spain and Latin America, examining the persistence of feudal and semi-feudal economic structures, social institutions and ideologies in these regions; the protracted nature of the physical and cultural struggle against this entrenched feudalism; the failure of both the liberal model of development and political democracy resulting in the preponderance of fascistic and monarchical regimes at the oligarchical level, and anarchist, trade-unionist, agrarian collectivist responses at the popular level, as well as other anti-liberal political formulations; a common confrontation with North American imperialism leading to political and cultural reactions in both (*Del Lazarillo* 17-18).

These structural similarities between Spanish and Latin American underdevelopment led to a mutual intellectual sympathy between certain sectors of the Spanish and Latin American intelligentsia. This relationship was in part occasioned by the European exile of a considerable number of Latin American intellectuals, including such figures as Rubén Darío, Alcides Arguedas, José Ingenieros, Francisco García Calderón, Manuel Ugarte, Rufino Blanco Fombona, José Santos Chocano and José Vasconcelos. Aside from fomenting a keen sense of group solidarity and pan-Americanism among these authors, the proximity to Spain brought about closer ties to kindred spirits among Spanish writers. Spanish journals such as *Germinal, Juventud, La vida literaria, Vida nueva, Revista nueva* and *La España moderna* formalized these ties by publishing the works of Latin American authors (Zuleta 44). Significantly, these journals were also the source of the dissemination of European degeneracy theory, publishing Spanish translations of and articles on authors such as Taine, Zola, Spencer and Nordau. Despite this intellectual cohabitation, there remained significant differences between the Spanish and Latin American literary groups owing to their different and multiple national origins and historical formations.

For the Spanish intellectuals of the turn-of-the-century, conventionally known as the *Generation of '98*, the discourse of national illness was the result of a centuries-long economic, political and cultural decadence painfully finalized by Spain's humiliating defeat by the United States in the Spanish-Cuban-American War of 1898. In addition to losing Spain's remaining colonies, the war symbolized what the Spanish intelligentsia constructed as a conflict between a modern, rational, Anglo-Saxon nation and a backwards, irrational Latin nation. Spain had lost, they reasoned, because of an interrelated racial, cultural and geographic inferiority which impeded modernization and manifested itself in psychopathologies such as the aboulia Ganivet diagnosed in the *Idearium español*. Not only did authors such as Ganivet label Spain as sick, they also conceived of themselves as socio-political "doctors." Ganivet refers to himself as a "médico espiritual" who will support his diagnosis with "casos clínicos." Nor was he the first or last Spaniard to address national underdevelopment in terms of collective illness. The following list gives an idea of the contemporary dissemination of this theme: Lucas Mallada, *Los males de la patria* (1890); Miguel de Unamuno, *En torno al casticismo* (1895); Ramón y Cajal, *Los tónicos de la voluntad* (1895); Pérez Pujol, *Historia de las instituciones sociales de la España goda* (1896); Ángel Ganivet, *Idearium español* (1897); Ricardo Macías Picavea, *El problema nacional* (1899); J. Martínez Ruiz, *El alma castellana* (1899); Rafael Altamira, *Psicología del pueblo español* (1902).

For Latin America, the economic and social progress associated with modernity was a utopian goal which was discursively invoked but concretely realized in a limited, fragmented and extremely unequal manner. Modernity's promise of an evolutionary transformation from pre-capitalist, semi-feudal, non-democratic societies to modern, industrialized liberal democracy was a promise which held true only for those hegemonic centers which modernized at the expense of colonialized peoples and peripheral regions whose economies were inserted into the international market in the dependent role of providing the raw materials for the center's compartmentalized needs. As François Perus has stated, "modernity" meant something entirely different in the Latin American context:

> Todo lo contrario: de la misma manera que la redefinición de las modalidades de inserción de América Latina en el sistema capitalista mundial llegado a su fase superior y última no podía convertir a los países del continente en naciones "desarrolladas",

puesto que se llevaba a cabo en el marco de la división internacional capitalista-imperialista de trabajo... (120)

In this sense, instead of undergoing a radical political and socio-
economic transformation at the end of the nineteenth century, Latin
America experienced a reconfiguration of its semi-feudal, *latifundista* organization in accordance with the requirements of the
global market.

At the ideological level, this gap between the discourse of
modernity and the reality of Latin America's insertion into the
world market placed the Latin American intelligentsia in a contradictory position. They were obliged to adopt a liberal, democratic,
market-based ideology that did not address the reality of Latin
American social, political and cultural institutions and that challenged their own class interests. The Latin American oligarchy generally was caught between the desire to acquire for itself the material benefits and cultural rhetoric of modernity and the unwillingness
or inability to square this material and cultural "progress" with political democracy and cultural recognition for the ethnically heterogeneous Latin American masses. The possibility of such political
and cultural inclusion also threatened the classist aesthetic sensibilities of oligarchical intellectuals of Latin American *modernismo* who
privileged the "high" European forms of written or learned culture
as opposed to popular oral or commercial mass culture (Beverley,
Literature 41).

In a partial attempt to rationalize this contradiction, certain segments of the Latin American intelligentsia appropriated the medical, psychological, ethnological and criminological discourse of degeneration employed by European intellectuals to explain the persistence of uneven development and marginality in their own societies. Carlos Octavio Bunge spoke of this application of modern
European degeneracy theory to the Latin American context in a letter to Alcides Arguedas praising the methodology of the latter's
Pueblo enfermo:

> Su estudio sobre el problema étnico es completo y sus conclu-
> siones me parecen acertadas. Estudia Ud. el tema con métodos
> europeos y con un criterio verdaderamente nacional. Ese me
> parece que debe ser el sistema de los sociólogos hispano-ameri-
> canos: utilizar la experiencia científica universal en beneficio
> propio nacional. (Roca 189)

Nevertheless, it is important to underline the perhaps obvious fact that the Latin American elite did not need to wait till the end of the nineteenth century to import an ideology capable of rationalizing the interdependent political, social, cultural and racial relations and practices in effect in Latin America since the time of its conquest and initial colonization. This fact was not lost on the Franco-Argentinean author Paul Groussac, a critic of social organicism in Latin America, who in 1896 stated: "La comparación de una sociedad con un organismo es más antigua que Spencer, Bacon, y el mismo Aristóteles..." (Stabb 34). The proto-scientific notion of pure blood introduced by the Spanish, the doctrine of "limpieza de sangre," together with the moral, juridical and scientific debate between the theological defenders of the indigenous populations, such as las Casas, and the "Aristotelian," "scientific" detractors, such as Sepúlveda, had laid the ideological grounds for an elaborate, hierarchical system of social and racial differentiation long before the arrival of the Social Darwinists.[5] It is also ironic to note that much of the new scientific thought produced in Europe in the nineteenth century relied on documentation from the Spanish colonies.

Yet the transformation of the requirements of the European hegemonic centers together with the concomitant process of nation building in newly independent Latin American nations demanded a scientific modernization of Latin America's previous discourses and practices of elite social legitimization. This simultaneous need to rationalize the perpetuation of colonial race relations and to reconfigure the *latifundista* economy led to the Spencerian formulations of social organicist thought in Latin America. These precursors to Latin American degeneracy theory argued that the rational development of national infrastructure and the correction of racial inferiority through immigration, genocide and education would place Latin America on the path to modernity. In both *Facundo* (1845) and *Conflicto y harmonia en las razas* (1883) the author-statesman

---

[5] It is interesting to note that Rafael de Altamira, in his *Psicología del pueblo español*, credits Sepúlveda with developing one of the first formulations of the Spanish national character or psychology. For a detailed discussion of the role of discovery myths and colonial ideological polemics in the formation of the eurocentric "scientific" conception of the Americas and its inhabitants, see Antonello Gerbi, *The Dispute of America*, trans. Jeremy Moyle (Pittsburgh: Univ. of Pittsburgh Press, 1973).

Domingo Sarmiento planned Argentina's modernization through a combination of infrastructure development, educational reform, immigration and the subjugation if not elimination of indigenous and mixed-race populations.

Yet when the economic benefits, cultural enlightenment and social progress promised by the discourse of modernity failed to materialize, the scientific belief in evolution turned inward in search of internal organic deficiencies within the national physiognomy and psychology. This was the juncture where optimistic positivism was transformed into pessimistic degeneracy theory.

The sheer number of authors and essays which perceived national and pan-American underdevelopment as a manifestation of psychological and physiological illness reflects the distinct national cultures and political republics in Latin America and the urgency which was ascribed to their "problem." The following list of texts may be conceived of as indicative: José María Ramos Mejía, *La neurosis de los hombres célebres en la historia argentina* (1878); Agustín Álvarez, *Manual de patología política* (1899); César Zumeta, *Continente enfermo* (1899); Carlos Octavio Bunge, *Nuestra América* (1903) and *Principios de psicología individual y social* (1903); Fernando Ortiz, *Los negros brujos. Apuntes para un estudio de etnografía criminal* (1905); Manuel Ugarte, *Enfermedades sociales* (1905); Alcides Arguedas, *Pueblo enfermo* (1909); Salvador Mendieta, *La enfermedad de Centro-América* (1910); Francisco García Calderón, *Les démocraties de l'Amérique* (1912); José Ingenieros, *Sociología argentina* (1913).

An investigation of these texts reveals a broad range of conflicting political ideologies. To the right of the political spectrum there is the anti-democratic conservatism of Bunge or the fascism of Arguedas; to the left there is the bio-economism of Ingenieros's socialism which embraced evolutionism, medical-psychological sociology and criminology. Of particular interest is the study of criminal ethnography by the Cuban anthropologist and promoter of African studies in Cuba, Fernando Ortiz. In *Los negros brujos*, which was heavily influenced by the Italian criminologist-psychologist Cesare Lombroso, Ortiz linked homosexuality and opium abuse to enervation, attributing those vices to Chinese immigrants, and labeled the persistence of African religious and medical practices in Cuba as degenerate, delinquent and parasitical. Ortiz's study is itself a commentary on the role of medicine in modern society. What is at stake for Ortiz is the right of Western medicine to monopolize modes of treatment, criminalize African healing practices, and to ascribe to itself the social, political and cultural authority, as is evident in this passage from *Los negros brujos* on voodoo:

> En todo caso, cuando la hechicería de los brujos prepara *embós*, tengan ó no acción real sobre el organismo humano, ello constituye un ejercicio ilegal de la medicina, y desde este punto de vista excuso patentizar la anti-socialidad de aquélla porque salta a la vista. Y la medicina bruja no sólo se extiende á los negros; bastantes blancos son sus víctimas, lo que prueba su arraigo y temebilidad. (363)

This cohabitation of different political ideologies within the discourse of national illness debunks our comfortable, present day notion that degeneracy theory was the intellectual drug of racist political troglodytes or self-loathing Europhiles. While this characterization of degeneracy theory is quite fitting in some cases, it does not encompass the full scope of evolutionary, raciological, psychological and medical discourse operating at the turn-of-the-century. In some instances, as in the case of Ortiz, degeneracy theory was the founding discourse of the "liberal" or progressive social sciences, while in others it was an instrument for conservative, or reactionary thought.

Adding to the disillusion with the promise of national progress was the emerging awareness that in some instances, the forces of modernity were antithetical to Latin American autonomy and cultural values. This twofold anxiety was heightened by the North American intervention of 1898. With the United States' acquisition of Cuba, Puerto Rico and the Philippines, the ambivalent ramifications of modernity for Latin America, which had already troubled José Martí before 1898, went on to concern intellectuals such as Manuel Ugarte, Rubén Darío, José Enrique Rodó and the innumerable authors associated with the *arielist* movement triggered by Rodó's *Ariel*. These authors reacted to the threat of an alien, imposed modernity at the national and pan-American level. For them, the imposition of a foreign, Anglo-Saxon modernity threatened to vulgarize Latin American cultural sensibilities with what they saw as the plebeian, commercial, sexually promiscuous and utilitarian culture of North American capitalism. Yet whereas Rodó's critique of the North American model in *Ariel* is limited to abstract, theoretical concerns about utilitarianism, Martí's direct experience of life in the United States resulted in a critique of specific mass culture phenomena, such as his abhorrence for the sort of mass entertainment of Coney Island and his discomfort in New York's streets which led him to medicalize the city as "este espléndido pueblo enfermo" (Ramos 151). Moreover, the threat of this intrusion was both politically external to Latin America, in the guise of political-military intervention, and internal to Latin America, reflecting a concern for Latin America's "youthful" spiritual, moral and psychological vulnerability to the crude, material appeal of the North American model.

In response to this menace, Martí, Rodó and Ugarte examined the "health" of America in the same fashion and using the same "scientific" criteria employed by pessimists like Bunge and Arguedas. However, unlike the racial pessimists, these authors also challenged the veracity or incurability of the medical diagnosis, either denying it outright as did Martí or by postulating an evolutionary cure as did Rodó and the *arielists*. In *Nuestra América* (1891), Martí criticized the shoddy application of science to racial diversity in the Americas, stating in a well-known phrase: "No hay batalla entre la civilización y la barbarie, sino entre la falsa erudición y la naturaleza" (39). In *Enfermedades sociales* Ugarte questioned whether the physiological and psychological deficiencies attributed to the Latin race were not in effect universal problems of underdevelopment:

> Debiéramos empezar por preguntarnos si realmente existe una raza latina y si los vicios y los yerros que advertimos en las naciones que con más o menos razón reclaman de ese origen, no son vicios y yerros universales, que nuestro meridonismo ha acentuado quizá, pero que se advierten en todas las naciones y no respetan las fronteras caprichosas en que algunos los quieren encerrar. (17)

In *Ariel*, Rodó shifted the onus of degeneracy away from Latin America and onto the supposed torchbearer of reason and progress, the United States. For Rodó, the deficiencies of Latin America were not exactly racial, but rather developmental, related to the continent's "immaturity." Yet, as I will argue, social organicism, evolutionism and moral degeneration surrounding the concept of cultural maturity betray a discourse rooted in the theories of racial and sexual enervation.

For an investigation of the discourse of national degeneration in Spain and Latin America, the significance of such thinkers as Ganivet and Unamuno in Spain, and Rodó and Ugarte in Latin America is that they introduced a degree of scientific and idealist skepticism into the consideration of national health. In this sense the various manifestations and responses to degeneration theory cannot be simply equated with positivism. On the contrary, in the *Idearium español* Ganivet attacks the fact-based blindness of science and impugns positivism by name. In *En torno al casticismo* Unamuno offers the following critique of the subjectivity of the "scientific method": "Y decimos algo, porque la ciencia no se da nunca pura, porque la geometría, y más que ella la química y muchísimo más la filosofía lleva algo en sí de precientífico, de sub-científico, de sobrecientífico como se quiera, de intracientífico en realidad, y este algo va teñido de materia nacional" (20). In Latin America, Rodó (and his followers) sought to correct what they saw as the vulgar instrumentality of science by returning it to a lofty, ideal, Socratic level, enabling them to disassociate themselves and Latin America from the material and cultural excesses of scientific progress while retaining its intellectual and ideal rigor. His program for cultural self-development and renewal through a scientific yet spiritually and morally pure education among male youth became a dominant model for decades throughout Latin America.

Starting from close readings of *Idearium español, Ariel,* and *Pueblo enfermo* (with supplementary examples from other Spanish and Latin American essays), I propose to map out the operation of the inter-related discourses of idealist aesthetics, evolutionism and medical and psychological pathology which inform these and other Spanish and Latin American essays of national identity. Through a deconstruction of the theoretical rhetoric of these texts, and by analyzing key intertextual references and comparing them with the seminal scientific and allied philosophical works of the period, I plan to show the dependence of such fundamental concepts as "national spirit," "genius," "ideals" and "character" on evolutionary science, a medical model of the male body and the accompanying mixed philosophical and anthropological psychiatry of the period.

In this sense I propose to trace the underlying connections between three specific genealogies of the discourse of illness in the turn-of-the-century Spanish and Latin American essay as opposed to undertaking an overview of a series of texts. I do so for the following reasons. First, I do not conceive of this investigation as a work of literary history or taxonomy. In this investigation I do not endeavor to systematically categorize essays as belonging or not belonging to a specific school of thought. In effect, I have countered this approach by juxtaposing texts which classic literary history has assigned to different literary traditions, movements and periods. My reading of *Idearium español*, *Ariel* and *Pueblo enfermo* cuts across more than one firmly established critical convention.

First, I compare the work of a Spaniard with that of two of his Latin American contemporaries. There is a body of solid scholarship which has compared these two traditions in the turn-of-the-century period. However, the bulk of this work has centered on a comparison of the aesthetics and themes of the Spanish Generation of '98 with that of Latin American *modernismo*. Despite the richness of this work, I have not sought to ground my investigation in these conventions of literary history. Rather, I examine the recurring metaphor or discourse of decadent national identity, a discourse which argues for a historically simultaneous shift to medical and psychological imagery in Spain and Latin America at the end of the nineteenth century. By thoroughly comparing specific textual instances of the Spanish and Latin American deployment of this discourse, I seek to substantiate the similar discursive structure and epistemological philology informing these texts.

Secondly, my study addresses three texts of vastly different ideology and political intention. In recognition of these differences, many critics have placed them in different, if not opposing, "positivist," "spiritualist" or "*modernista*" camps. Indeed, the juxtaposition of the conservative, eccentric thought of Ángel Ganivet with that of an enlightened liberal such as José Enrique Rodó, in the company of the vehemently racist and pessimistic invective of Alcides Arguedas, is provocative. I intend it to be so. By situating the conventionally labeled "positivist" thought of Arguedas with what has been traditionally characterized as Ganivet's and Rodó's "spiritual" reaction against positivism, I intend to show how the psychological, evolutionary and medical imagery which characterizes the discourse of illness transcended political ideology and intention in the turn-of-the-century period.

This last point leads us back to questions of strategy or method. Inasmuch as my study juxtaposes texts in ways which contradict established critical cannons, it has been incumbent upon me to ac-

quire the theoretical tools necessary to substantiate my argument.
The overriding issue here is one of evidence. Literary criticism
within the discipline of hispanism about these texts has tended to
reproduce the approaches concerning literary periods, movements
and biographies in a specific political context. There have been
striking exceptions to which I am indebted. Specifically, with regard to the discourse of illness in Spain and Latin America, I am indebted to two classic, seminal works, H. Ramsden's *The 1898
Movement in Spain. Towards a Reinterpretation with Special Reference to* En torno al casticismo *and* Idearium español; and Martin
Stabb's *In Quest of Identity. Patterns in the Spanish American Essay
of Ideas, 1890-1960.* Among other things, Ramsden's work is particularly useful in tracing Ganivet's thought to that of the French theorist Hippolyte Taine, while Stabb provides a masterful overview of
the pessimistic theoreticians of Latin American degeneracy such as
Arguedas.

Nevertheless, when I initially read *Idearium español, Ariel* and
Pueblo enfermo, I was aware that these were texts which lay beyond the reach of standard literary criticism. The many studies
which examined these texts did not thoroughly address the "non-
literary" discourses of natural selection, psychology, criminology,
sexology, and medicine operating in these essays. The exceptions
which did discuss the notion of the sick nation have done so by ad-
dressing the political or social ideas of conservatives and overt
racists. What has not been investigated up to this point, in my esti-
mation, is the language or rhetoric of national illness, not as an idea,
but as a grammar inflected by notions of race, evolution and gender, a grammar which is spoken throughout the political spectrum.

In order to verify my reading of the discourse of degeneration I
have had to familiarize myself with the contemporary treatises in
these fields. Furthermore, to better understand these texts I have
had recourse to current advances in the study of discourse, feminist
theory, queer theory, cultural studies and art history. This new theoretical work, particularly in the area of discourse and gender, has
complemented the knowledge acquired from the many exceptional
works within hispanism on these texts.

Finally, in order to conclusively assert the presence of an epistemological continuity in these disparate texts, I feel that a systematic
and rigorous analysis of the rhetoric of illness is required. It is one
thing to state that given texts share an idea, or, in this case, are in-

formed by a shared discourse of illness. Yet it is quite another thing to give evidence of this assertion through textual analysis. In this instance I believe that the process of analysis is just as significant as the conclusions. Inasmuch as I am attempting to map-out the different sexual, racial, political and social workings of the discourse of illness in turn-of-the-century Spain and Latin America, especially in texts which I have chosen for their ideological dissonance, the decision to concentrate primarily on the three texts previously noted seems to me a prudent one. I will leave it to the reader to decide whether I have been successful in this objective.

CHAPTER 1

ÁNGEL GANIVET'S *IDEARIUM ESPAÑOL* AND
THE MODEL OF NATIONAL ILLNESS

REPRESSION AND DENIAL

Ángel Ganivet's *Idearium español* documents the intellectual-psychological struggle of the author upon finding himself surrounded and interpellated by the inter-related effects of Spain's decline as an imperial power and of capitalist modernization and industrialization, an unfolding process of socio-historical change which he, and his contemporaries, experienced as a kind of spiritual and somatic malaise or degeneration. Ganivet categorizes this trauma of social adaptation as a crisis of the human spirit or condition, a crisis which he goes on to interpret in medical and psychological terms.

The *Idearium español* (1897) is neither the first nor the only text to perceive "el problema de España" in the terms of psychosomatic character illness. Lucas Mallada's *Los males de la patria* (1890), Unamuno's *En torno al casticismo* (1895), Ramón y Cajal's *Los tónicos de la voluntad* (1895), Pérez Pujol's *Historia de las instituciones sociales de la España goda* (1896) and Rafael Altamira's *Psicología del pueblo español* (1902) also consider Spain's concrete historical circumstances within the medical-spiritual paradigm.

Part of what distinguishes the *Idearium español* is the degree to which it mixes this analysis of Spain's political, economic and spiritual health with a discourse of personal confession and self-diagnosis. Despite the cultural-spiritual seclusion of the *Idearium español*, there are psychological, political and aesthetic, that is, *ideological*, residues of discourses which escape its self-reflexive idealism. This confluence of the personal and the national informs both the theoretical premises and the methodology employed by the text as well as the narrative or anecdotal content. This intersection of the boundaries between the obsessively autobiographic and the methodological and thematic collapse of the subject-object opposition are central to the *Idearium español* specifically, and are also inherent, in a more general sense, to the critical project of the subsequent Generation of '98. As H. Ramsden has stated: "The prober of national destinies is no longer a mere observer; the subject and object of study are fused; knowledge henceforth is involvement, necessity, anguish" (*Idearium* 82).

Ganivet addresses Spain's national *anguish*, which is in reality a crisis of transformation, its decline from a colonial power to an underdeveloped nation; and from a pre-industrial to an industrial society. Along with these concrete macrosocial changes, Ganivet confronts the transformation of social relations, the alienating effects of mechanization and commercialization on daily life and the deep psychological, spiritual and ontological shifts that these changes entail. Ganivet wrote the *Idearium español* as a spiritual biography (or as many have argued, autobiography) of Spain. The narrative modality of this national profile constantly switches between a self-interested medical diagnosis, a subjective philosophy of territorial determinism, purely personal commentaries on historical events, and autobiographic anecdotes of illustrative encounters from Ganivet's life. The resulting mixture is a profoundly personal treatise on the national character, with Ganivet offering or exposing himself as a prime example.

Thus, at one level, the *Idearium español* functions as a pathogenesis of Spain and its intelligentsia (including Ganivet). But, as has been mentioned, the text mobilizes many discourses, including the philosophical, the psychological and the theological, employing them in a highly subjective, if not autobiographical register. This leads to curious and provocative images and discussions which do not exactly fit the conscious subject-object fusion of the text, namely Ganivet-Spain, intelligentsia-nation, doctor-patient, diagnosis-illness, to suggest another level of discursive self-cure or confession with regard to disturbances of a more personal, intimate or libidinal nature. That is to say that the text resounds with *anguish* and preoccupations other than the spiritual and material state of Spain and its people, and that these non-national and personal associations cofunction with and within the stated purpose of the text, the spiritual regeneration of Spain.

It is this personal anguish which recurs as a kind of negated absent cause and which is sublimated into the very fabric of *Idearium español*'s national proposal. Nevertheless, as with any other mental or ideological projection or representation, the underlying but sublimated referent of the text contains the traces of its original conception and occlusion. Through an examination of this trace of the original idea, it is possible to reconstruct the text's greater context of conceptual associations and affiliations, – what Unamuno called the "nimbo" of the idea. Or in the case of the *Idearium español*, to remove what Ganivet terms as the "hoja de parra del senequismo."

The ideological distancing between Ganivet and his immediate social environment originates, in part, with his refusal to recognize the role of culture in the reproduction of the relations and conditions of social and economic production. Ganivet denies the material roots of culture. This denial of social transformation is conceptually linked to his repression of specific personal associations concerning the body, the material and history. The *Idearium español*'s basis in chaste idealism and transcendental territorial determinism denies that culture registers humanity's attempts at surviving, controlling and dominating nature. [6] In a contradictory two step process, Ganivet clearly associates the social reorganization of life under capitalism with decay, only to negate the importance of such superficial changes for the pure, eternal national spirit. Ganivet initiates a materialist analysis and critique of culture and then represses it. Thus, despite Ganivet's intention, the *Idearium español* is a cultural instrument which represents, expresses and *realizes* its capacity and will to reproduce and control its environment through the reciprocal functions of representation and practice. It is the testimony of an individual's attempt to organize the rule of a nation and himself.

It is this dynamic relation between culture and the social, together with economic and political practices (or perhaps a specific alignment of these under capitalist democracy) that horrifies

---

[6] This idea is derived from my reading of Adorno's "Spengler After the Decline" from *Prisms*. As Adorno affirms, Spengler disconnects human history from nature. Within this vision, the ongoing struggle to subjugate nature is situated outside of the human conscience. History is posited as an *intra-history* closed to the material world inasmuch as the former is tied to the supposed constancy of the human spirit. The immutability of the spirit or soul of intra-history negates the possibility of changing the human condition.

Ganivet. For Ganivet, the mediation between culture and social practice constitutes the degeneration of the former. The social isolation of the pure Spanish soul postulated in the *Idearium español*, elevates culture above the vulgar and common affairs of civil society, and in an analogous movement, above the body. In order to humanize culture, Ganivet removes it from contact with both the social and anatomical body.[7]

This profound contradiction of Ganivet, where his intention of humanizing culture in fact makes it more abstract and mechanical, arises from the psychological dilemma of the author as an individual and national voice. The conceptual disjuncture between thought and action, culture and civilization, mind and body, paralyzes the text, either ingraining the nation in an immutable territorial destiny or resigning it to a passive, victimized role in world affairs. The mechanical determinism employed in the text leaves no other option than to follow the prescription of a territorial personality and to adhere to a social planning based on this hermeneutics of spirit. According to this vision, to reflect upon the national future outside the bounds of the spiritual diagnosis is to engage in a project condemned to historical anemia, an illness that the *Idearium español* seeks to cure.

Ganivet's philosophical fatalism is related to the conflict between his ideological interpellation and his psychic existence. Specifically, between his immersion in an increasingly rationalized and commercialized society and the way in which his resistance to this capitalist modernization was complemented and reinforced by prior internal conflicts of subject formation. Ganivet's ideological-intellectual will to repress the sensual-corporal (or material-historical) aspect constitutes the conceptual and physical opposition which motivates the text. In the *Idearium español* this conflict is manifest respectively and inter-dependently in a series of oppositions which contrast the qualities ascribed to the true Spanish essence to the superficial, degenerate or imposed qualities of modernity. The central oppositions are: the ideal vs. the material,

---

[7] As Adorno points out in "Cultural Criticism and Society," the ideological self-absorption of bourgeois culture originates in the denial of the connections between culture and socio-economic practice. The role that culture plays in the reproduction and enforcing of the social relations of production is denied. Bourgeois culture withdraws into itself, proclaiming a purity from the inequality which surrounds it.

the sensual vs. the chaste, the mind vs. the body, the interior vs. the exterior, the healthy vs. the sick, the territorial vs. the historical, the symbolic vs. the real, the traditional vs. the modern, use value vs. exchange value.

The tension between the socio-cultural prescriptions of the second half of the nineteenth century and individual libidinal expressions is certainly not exclusive to Ganivet. The literature, philosophy and indeed the very "science" of sexuality, and the emerging discipline of psychology of the period are characterized by obsessions concerning gender, the sensual or sexual. The *Idearium español*, notwithstanding its pretensions to spiritual chastity, is clearly situated within this preoccupation with the sexual. In fact, within the very binary oppositions which seek to repress or devalue the sexual, we observe a curiously negative emphasis on the links between the sexual and the spiritual, the ideal and the material. We must therefore consider the function of repression in the *Idearium español* in this light, not as an act of absolute exclusion, repugnance or censure, but one of channeling, displacement and regimentation. This passage from Michel Foucault's *The History of Sexuality* underscores this point:

> There is no binary division to be made between what one says and what one does not say; we must try to determine the different ways of not saying such things, how those who can and those who cannot are distributed, which type of discourse is authorized, or which form of discretion is required in any case. (27)

In the *Idearium español* the authorized voices are those of the doctor-psychologist and the philosopher-priest, both of whom are empowered to say that which cannot be said, to repress the very discourse which they pronounce. Yet, the text includes the voice of the patient and the confessor who at times merge into the respective figures of the sick doctor or the confessing priest reminiscent of Unamuno's *San Manuel Bueno, mártir*.

In turn-of-the-century Spain, sexual *ethos*, or in other words, the discursive and social distribution and regimentation of sexuality, formed a decisive component of the relations and mode of production. For Ganivet, Unamuno and other writers of the period, this internalized psycho-sexual formation acquired a parallel signification in the national debate surrounding economic development and colonial expansion. The concrete factors of the exterior world, material scarcity, biological limitations and cultural coercion coincide to restrict the free expression of the sexuality of the individual, an internalized and individualized interpellation that is subsequently returned to the collective forum in the form of a sexually charged socio-political ideology which equates chastity with national purity. In this way material and social forces inscribe themselves in the individual and collective imaginary and are thus reproduced materially and *imaginarily*. From this operation of the sexual interpellation of the subject arises: 1) the conflict between an individual's desires and the cultural rules of society; 2) the projection of this internalized conflict onto broader social and national issues. The sexual ideology of the individual and his/her social constituency comes out of this double process. As with any instance of ideological interpellation, sexual ideology results from the imaginary distancing of an individual from the real conditions of his/her existence. In this case, the disjuncture between the real possibilities of *eros* and the discourses and practices permitted by society on one hand, and the sublimation of this gap into the competing isolationist and integralist models of national development on the other.

The form and perception of the process is historically conditioned by the economic, political and cultural circumstances of the moment. As in the case of the interpellation of national subjects, this process of the sexual/social formation of the individual is an implosive movement. The sexual interpellation of the subject becomes a phenomenon of privatized, introspective and closed reflection. In the *Idearium español*, this movement of psycho-sexual withdrawal, posited as the origin of the true disinterested ideal, is simultaneously applied as a political philosophy of economic and political seclusion. But the psychic internalization of the dialectic between the individual and society, mimicked in the spiritual and material internalization of national policy, leaves behind the extra-personal and international traces of a forced interiorization. There is no concept or aesthetic work which exhausts itself in itself, in its pure existence. Art and philosophy develop in relation to the real and historical conditions of their moment.

The psychic interiorization of ideology points to another stage in the human conquest of nature. In the *Idearium español* the postulate of the pure and ahistorical national soul indicates the domination of desire. The rupture between human conscience and its concrete social environment announces the artificial divorce between mind and body. The mind becomes an autonomous and eternal entity, completely resistant to historical-material corruption. The body becomes the vessel of history, vulnerable to the brutality, arbitrariness and vulgarity of material production and distribution and the political system which accompanies them. In Ganivet's passionate denial of the connections between the national spirit and its material context, precisely the opposite is implied. His emotional separation of the material-sensual-historical *continuum* from the spiritual-aesthetic-ideal suggests an uncomfortable recognition of the same. That is, such an attempt seeks to deny that which concerns it the most.

The sexual repression which underlies the *Idearium español*'s spiritual philosophy and national policy becomes clearer if we consider Ganivet's notion of the disinterested and chaste ideal. Significantly, apart from terms which define the ideal in clearly sexually charged terms of warrior-chastity (*puro, cristiano, estoico, religioso, conquistador*), and hygiene (*limpio, sin mancha*), there is a third category which designates this spiritual-national purity in spatial terms (*alto, elevado*). This spatial metaphor is associated with non-partisan, judicious political insight: "pero no encontraremos uno solo que vea y juzgue la política nacional desde un punto de vista elevado..." (*IE* 115). Yet how does this spatial relationship confer purity and chastity on "lo elevado?" A genealogy of the "elevated" or the "high" leads us back to the division of the body into upper and lower halves. The former is symbolized by the head, which looks up to the fixed celestial spheres and the perfect origin of the universe, God. Contrasted to this are the genitals and feet, the "low" parts which face the earth and all the "base" creatures who walk upon on all fours. Freud has characterized this sublimated division of the body into a spatially divided ideal of the "high" and "low" in the following way:

> It is to the effect that, with the assumption of an erect posture by man and with the depreciation of his sense of smell, it was not only his anal erotism which threatened to fall victim to organic repression, but the whole of his sexuality; so that since this, the sexual function has been accompanied by a repugnance which cannot further be accounted for, and which prevents its complete satisfaction and forces it away from the sexual aim into sublimations and libidinal displacements. (59)

The *Idearium español* offers ample evidence of this psycho-social association between spatial descent into the sexual region of the body as a symbolic short-hand for social and political decadence. An obsession or repugnance for the sexual function is linked to a critique of materialism and the inescapable corruption of the political application of ideas:

> Y pienso que así se nos presentan las ideas, las cuales empiezan por un destello divino que, conforme toma *cuerpo* en la realidad, va perdiendo su originaria *pureza*, hasta *hundirse* y *encenegarse* en las más groseras *encarnaciones*. Por un instante que el alma se deleite en la contemplación de una idea que nace *limpia* y sin *mancha* entre las espumas del pensamiento, ¡cuánta angustia después para hacer sensible esa idea en alguna de las menguadas y *raquíticas* formas de nuestro escaso poder dispone, cuánta tristeza al verla convertida en algo *material*, *manchada* por la *impureza* inseparable de lo *material*! (my italics 88)

In this passage we observe the ambiguous nature of Ganivet's "national" preoccupation and what is at the origin of his own heart-felt "tristeza." His anguish comes out of the association of materiality with physical descent ("hundirse") into the lower sexual half of the body ("toma cuerpo," "encarnaciones"), a region he associates with filth ("encenegarse," "manchada") and degenerative illness ("raquíticas"). It is the reality of the body, of sexuality which saddens him. This sexual repression is projected onto the nation in the sphere of the material, causing a lamentable but unavoidable ("inseparable") "impureza."

Idearium español's vision of a chaste territorial spirit as the true motivating force of the national ideal, in reality a displaced program for national empowerment, manifests his contempt for the real conditions of his existence, first in terms of the repression of desire and the body and secondly in terms of the denial of a process of social modernization and industrialization already in effect. The abstract separation from the real world which Ganivet affects is his way of dealing with it. In this way the sexual component of ideology reproduces the distorted and imaginary relation of the individual to reality. The sexual interpellation of the individual and society is disseminated in culture and reproduced in individual consciousness. In Ganivet's *Idearium español*, the sexual and gender based model of subject formation takes on a broader role of social interpellation, grounding the issues of domestic and foreign policy in a sexually inflected discourse. The thematic and discursive association between corporeality, sexuality and history is omnipresent in its conspicuous and ongoing negation. In the introspective and repressive illusion of the text, concrete, historical reality, the bodily manifestations of the socio-political, are replaced by a repressed and asexual mythology of Spain.

SPAIN AS VIRGIN

Ganivet reveals the psychic connections between sexuality and history in the repressive symbolization with which he begins the *Idearium español*:

> Muchas veces, reflexionando sobre el apasionamiento con que en España ha sido defendido y proclamado el dogma de la Concepción Inmaculada, se me ha ocurrido pensar que en el fondo de ese dogma debía de haber algún misterio que por ocultos caminos se enlazara con el misterio de nuestra alma nacional; que acaso ese dogma era el símbolo, ¡símbolo admirable!, de nuestra propia vida, en la que, tras larga y penosa labor de maternidad, venimos a hallarnos a la vejez con el espíritu virgen; como una mujer que, atraída por irresistible vocación a la vida monástica y ascética y casada contra su voluntad y convertida en madre por deber, llegara al cabo de sus días a descubrir que su espíritu era ajeno a su obra, que entre los hijos de la carne el alma continuaba sola, abierta como una rosita mística a los ideales de la virginidad. (9)

The symbolic comparison between Spain and the Virgin Mary underlines several foundations of the religious-psychological and spiritual-sensual formation of the text. This image works through the same model of spatial, corporal and hygienic descent previously noted with regard to Ganivet's sense of the corruption of the ideal, only in this instance it is the national spirit which experiences the "tristeza de verla convertida en algo material," or in other words, of entering into socio-economic and material history. Yet unlike the corruption of the ideal, the territorial spirit, although violated, remains pure and is not "manchada por la impureza inseparable de lo material." Spain is forced into material history but is essentially impervious to the same.

Ganivet explicitly links this notion of national purity to sexual innocence in *El Porvenir de España*, where he defends his mistaken application of the dogma of the Immaculate conception:

> El dogma de la Inmaculada Concepción se refiere, es cierto, al pecado original, pero al borrar este último pecado da a entender la suma pureza y santidad. El dogma literal se presta además a esa amplia interpretación, porque las palabras "concebida sin mancha" dicen al alma del pueblo español dos cosas: que la Virgen *fue concebida* sin mancha, y que *es concebida* sin mancha eternamente por el espíritu humano. Hay el hecho de la concepción real, y el fenómeno de la concepción ideal por el hombre de una mujer que, no obstante haber vivido vida humana, se vio libre de la mancha que la materia imprime a los hombres. (196)

Original sin, namely human sexuality, particularly female sexuality, is erased or repressed (*borrar*), an act of repression which is clearly associated here with the denial of Spain's colonial past and its contemporary confrontation with liberal democracy and capitalism. Yet it is significant in and of itself that this political metaphor is located within the body of a woman who has given birth but who has had no active role in the conception or rearing of the child. Spain is posited as a woman who has lived but not in any recognizably human way, a woman who has left no material or subjective trace and who exists in a kind of mystic, transcendental fog. It is man, both in the guise of the Holy Spirit and history, who transgresses this mystical virginity. Masculine political and intellectual agency is identified with sexual agency, and both in turn are stabilized by a feminine passivity which obeys a more profound mythological, territorial wisdom or *intrahistoria*. In this way the notion of feminine passivity or non-subjectivity exercises a unifying, transhistorical function throughout the vicissitudes of national history. As Matías Montes Huidobro explains, in Ganivet:

> Los ascensos y descensos históricos, los momentos de grandeza y de decadencia, dirigidos por empresas masculinas, resultan estabilizados por la pasividad femenina. En las etapas de corrupción es la mujer, blanca y dúctil, el vehículo de soborno. Pero siempre mantiene su virginidad espiritual dentro de su permanencia histórica. (16)

The simile of Spain as virgin brings into play different conceptual associations concerning the psycho-sexual formation of the individual, female sexuality and reproduction, and mysticism. And as the simile itself proclaims, the complex psychological, religious and sexual connotations of the doctrine of the Immaculate Conception, which Ganivet has confused with the concept of the virgin-birth, are now projected onto the social, economic and cultural problems confronting Spain in the late nineteenth century.

The combination of maturity and youth in a single image is a classic *topos* of pagan and Christian antiquity (Curtius 101). The importance of this image in the *Idearium español* situates Ganivet within the Spanish *fin de siècle* affinity for the Middle Ages and medieval allegory.[8] Spain, however, was not the only nation to be represented by medieval figures in the nineteenth century. Other idealized medieval virgins such as Britannia and Germania functioned in a similar way to the *Idearium español*'s Virgin Mary, representing eternal, pre-industrial values of purity and chastity, serving as a kind of moral shield against the ills of modernity (Mosse 98). The application of this *topos* in the *Idearium español* ("venimos a hallarnos a la vejez con el espíritu virgen") corresponds to the discursive intersection of theology and the discipline of psychology with the social imaginary of the *fin-de-siècle* period. The figure of the Virgin combines two impossible and parallel phenomena in a homologous identity: a virgin mother; a nation without history. As a political metaphor, it explains that Spain's virginal spirit was violated by imperial expansion, forcing her into a maternal relationship (with the colonies) for which she had no vocation. With this symbol Ganivet negates Spanish history as an external transgression. In fact, according to the text's depiction of a forced maternity, Spanish history constitutes a violation of its national soul or essence.

The notion of the Spanish spirit's virginity denies or represses two conceptually linked material-physical realities inimical to the *Idearium español*. First it denies the long history of Spain's imperial rise and fall and its subsequent socio-economic and cultural transformation under capitalism. Secondly it denies or represses sexuality, in this specific instance female sexuality (yet as we shall see the

---

[8] For a discussion of Medievalism in nineteenth century Spanish literature see Lily Litvak, *A Dream of Arcadia: Anti-Industrialism in Spanish Literature* (Austin and London: Univ. of Texas Press, 1975).

concept of spiritual virginity is extended to the male as well in the figure of Seneca, a non-sexual male).

Ganivet has left behind contradictory statements regarding his opinion of women's character and role in society. There would seem to be many persona in him, one being the public social reformer, another being the favorite child of an exceedingly devoted mother, another that of an embittered partner in a tumultuous and often unhappy sexual relationship. In the final article of his series on Granada published in 1896, Ganivet championed the inclusion of women in Spain's cultural, professional and commercial life. Influenced by the social integration of women in Helsinki where he had been in the diplomatic service Ganivet wrote: "En suma: el sexo es un accidente que no influye más que en el vestir y en la elección de algunos oficios que por su naturaleza exigen, ya la delicadeza de la mujer, ya la fuerza del hombre" (*Granada* 88). Yet it should be mentioned that even this voice of social reform distinguished between independent, single, professional women and married women, whose role Ganivet limited to the preservation of the family.

Contrasted to this conditionally positive public voice of feminine inclusion, Ganivet's personal correspondence expresses a bitter and hostile attitude towards women. This private and negative side of Ganivet's view of women was perhaps tied to the problems of mutual infidelity and distrust which plagued him and his mistress, Amelia Roldán. In a letter he wrote from Belgium we see the negation of female subjectivity and the construction of a purely symbolic femininity reminiscent of the repressive image of the Virgin. Ganivet stated that:

> Delante de la hija de Eva que tira coces y huele, y no a ámbar, no queda más vía libre que la del hidalgo manchego ante la moza tobosina: tomar de ella la "idea de sexo" nada más (el olor, como quien dice), y reconstruir sobre este pequeño cimiento un castillo imaginario que llegue hasta donde se pueda. Dentro de ese castillo es donde únicamente puede habitar la señora de nuestros pensamientos, la que nos inspire un amor que sea algo distinto del usual y corriente entre los animales. (*Obras* 2: 971)

As with the image of Spain as the Virgin Mary, this symbolic reduction of women denies their subjectivity through an erasure of female sexuality. In this vehemently misogynist passage, sexuality,

specifically female sexuality, is associated with olfactory unpleas-
antness and animals in a way which prefigures Freud's description
cited above of the negative, repressive association between the concept of original sin ("la hija de Eva"), the olfactory sense, the pejo-
ratively perceived "animal" nature of human sexuality and the spatial metaphor of the "high" and the "low." Here Ganivet suggests
another basis for "spiritual" union between men and women; one
based on the repression of female sexuality and, in a larger sense,
subjectivity. He is close here to his Austrian contemporary Otto
Weininger, who stated that women "must really and truly and spontaneously relinquish coitus. That undoubtedly means that woman,
as woman, must disappear..." (Dijkstra 220). Yet within this erasure
of female sexuality, a sublimated and mystic discourse of feminine
sexuality resurfaces in the sensual flower imagery which ends the
text's opening passage: "el alma continuaba sola, abierta como una
rosita mística a los ideales de la virginidad" (my italics). In this
sense sexuality is not completely repressed through omission but is
elevated through discursive displacement to a spiritual-mystical
plane.

Considering the close relationship between Ganivet and his
mother and the divinely maternal, symbolic and fictional image of
the Virgin which he so ardently champions, a kind of sublimated
and obsessive love of mother is not mere biographical speculation.
In fact, the *Idearium español* is not his only work which assigns a
national-allegorical function to the image of motherhood. In *trabajo*
IV of his novel *Los trabajos del infatigable creador Pío Cid* the
prayer to "Nuestra Madre" not only evokes an extremely conservative political and nostalgic view of pre-industrial Granada, but also
"lends itself to a psychoanalytic interpretation as the expression of
the author's longing for union with an omnipotent mother" (Ginsberg 101). In *Cartas finlandesas* Ganivet defines women's reason for
being in aesthetic-erotic-reproductive terms: "Una mujer deforma-
da por el exceso de la maternidad es más bella que un marimacho...
La belleza de la mujer está en su aptitud para vivir como mujer, y en
la obra que realiza como mujer" (Montes Huidobro 11). Here the
time-worn ideological cliche of maternal beauty is sustained with
decidedly back-handed compliments. The "deformed," pregnant
woman is more beautiful than any "tomboy" (marimacho) because
she is following her prescribed function. Her beauty resides in her
moral acquiescence to this reproductive role. As Montes Huidobro

has argued, the inter-relation between eroticism, reproduction, the grotesque and women's social function is central to Ganivet's work.[9] Throughout it, references to motherhood connote selfless altruism, as opposed to capitalist competition and utilitarianism; the erotically sublimated sexual-material chastity and innocence of the mother-child relationship merges with a *costumbrista* vision of Spain's pre-industrial virtue which becomes indistinguishable from autobiographical references to the author's childhood.

What is exceptional about the symbolic substitution-repression of sexuality and history is that it projects a mental phenomenon of the sexual-ideological distancing of a child from its mother onto the nation. The symbolization of Spain as the Virgin represents the social transference of a phenomenon particular to compulsive children, the doubt of one's legitimate origin. This anxiety concerning legitimacy is concisely articulated here in this citation from the early twentieth-century psychoanalyst Wilhelm Stekel:

> In no case of compulsion will this doubt in one's origin be missing. It may also be directed against the mother: "Am I a changeling, an adopted child?" This doubt leads to strong repressions in the sphere of fantasies; it leads to birth and womb fantasies... (*Compulsion* 1: 259)

The proposition of the absolute, ahistorical purity and chastity of the Spanish soul obscures the suspicion of a possibly impure origin and identity. The symbol of the Virgin represents the repression of its opposite, of corporeality, history, of the idea in its original scope of accepted and repressed associations.

This repression is the result of doubt and anxiety concerning identity, in the case of the *Idearium español*, the undifferentiated identity of Ganivet-Spain. The text seemingly mimics the classic psychoanalytic analysis of the compulsive child. Ganivet's obsession with the virginity of his nation/mother associates birth fantasies with national history. In the personal and national introspection or

---

[9] Regarding *La conquista del reino de Maya por el último conquistador español, Pío Cid*, Montes Huidobro states: "el erotismo como vehículo de fecundidad: las caderas; la cantidad como vehículo expresivo de la fecundidad: cuarenta hijos; lo grotesco como símbolo de fecundidad: el vientre de vaca; la transformación física como expresión de fecundidad: el pecho pequeño, que en lengua maya aparece designado como memé, convertido en grande por razones fisiológicas" (12).

infantile self-absorption of the text, sexuality and history conspire to violate the image of the Virgin-mother-nation, forcing her to endure the "vulgarity" and pain of childbirth and history. Yet as with the compulsive child, Ganivet denies this sexual-historical reality, anxiously doubting and proclaiming the purity of his mother-nation.

The relationship between the child and his/her parents, or Ganivet and Spain, acquires a contradictory tension of love and hate, trust and suspicion, acceptance and denial. Within this familial-national scenario or narrative, there develops an imaginary and distorted distance of the child from his/her parents, of the subject from its national interpellation. The child – Ganivet – is preoccupied with the chastity and fidelity of his/her parents-nation to the point of obsession. In the *Idearium español* fidelity is an amalgam of sexual-spiritual loyalty to the analogously chaste and economically disinterested territorial spirit. The child's perception of, and relation to the world is conditioned by this ideological break with his/her parents, as is Ganivet's perception of national decline and modernization, a break based on doubt about one's position in society and the power that this position provides. In the *Idearium español,* the suspicion of the legitimacy of the text's own undifferentiated identity and origins manifests a profound doubt and initiates the subsequent repression concerning personal and national identity. This uncertainty precipitates the necessity of repressing disturbing ideas and desires as well as denying national history and contemporary socio-historical processes.

In this psychoanalytic paradigm of subject formation we see the constitution of an ideology, that of oedipal differentiation from parents. The *Idearium español* leaves behind the traces of the repression of this process, inter-splicing its rejection of the corporal-sexual into its ascetic, anti-materialist and anti-modernization national proposal. In this way Ganivet reproduces the imaginary distancing from his own libidinal-corporeal conditions of existence at the macrosocial and political level, a social-sexual "distancia psicológica de la realidad española de su época" (Fox 27).

Seneca's Fig Leaf and the Medicalization of Sexuality

The figure of Seneca in *Idearium español* fulfills a similar function as the Virgin, denoting both introspective meditation and sexual chastity, as opposed to a dependence on foreign ideas and models of development which are associated with materialism and sexuality. As we can see in the following passage extolling the virtues of Senecan stoicism, this dichotomy is also related in spatial terms which oppose interior to exterior experience:

> No te dejes vencer por nada extraño a tu espíritu; piensa, en medio de los accidentes de la vida, que tienes dentro de ti una fuerza madre, algo fuerte e indestructible, como un eje diamantino, alrededor del cual giran los hechos mezquinos que forman la trama del diario vivir; y sean cuales fueren los sucesos que sobre ti caigan, sean de los que llamamos prósperos, o de los que llamamos adversos, o de los que parecen envilecernos con su contacto, mantente de tal modo firme y erguido, que al menos se pueda decir siempre de ti que eres un hombre. (46)

As Miguel Olmedo Moreno has pointed out, this may not be an accurate synopsis of stoicism, but it is certainly a strange and provocative summation of the national spirit (25). At the political level this pseudo-stoic motto repeats the principal ideas presented by the metaphor of the Virgin: Spain's true essence and hope of regeneration lies within its own national spirit and territorial character. Also like the image of the Virgin, the figure of Seneca is a decidedly pre-modern and pre-industrial symbol which seeks to lend a timeless immutability to the national character. But whereas the feminine ideal embodied in the Virgin remains allegorically passive, the virtues of virile manliness personified by Seneca represent the dynamic aspect of the national spirit. As George L. Mosse has argued, the nineteenth-century concept of manliness was crucial to the foundation of nationalist ideology. Manliness and male virtue guaranteed the control of the sexual instincts which both the sexologist Kraft-Ebing and the psychoanalyst Freud deemed necessary for the health of civilization. Manliness, or Senecan stoicism in the *Idearium español*, served as a bulwark against the effects of the social transformation of modernity, positing male virtue and virility as a reservoir of national health and vitality. [10]

The symbolic function of Seneca, or more precisely Ganivet's later reference to the Spanish spirit which "se cubre con la hoja de parra del senequismo," also establishes a repressive identity between the ideal and chastity. Of course it is Ganivet who has added this sexual dimension to Seneca, providing him with a fig-leaf and inscribing him into the code of sexual-historical virginity. It is an ambiguous gesture of sexual enhancement and repression which is central to the text, or as Michel Foucault has stated: "a refusal concerning the very thing that was brought to light and whose formulation was urgently solicited" (*History* 55).

A closer reading of the passage about Seneca reveals a model for sexual-political repression or abstinence based on fears of corporeal, mental, and national debilitation through social or sexual intercourse. The early mention of Seneca in the *Idearium español* inaugurates a discourse centered around the conservation or squandering of *energies*. In the late nineteenth century, scientists, "sexologists" and psychologists were obsessed with the loss of vitality through the "excessive" discharge of fluids during sexual activity. Such discharges of energy were thought to divert blood-flow from the brain, leaving the individual in a physically and mentally dissipated state. As one contemporary sexologist stated: "the frequent exercise of the act of copulation leads directly to anemia, malnutrition, asthemia of the muscles and nerves, and mental exhaustion" (Dijkstra 170).

Specifically in the case of the *Idearium español*, the intertextual "scientific" concern for energy and its conservation comes from the work of the French philosopher-naturalist Alfred Fouillée. The writings of Fouillée, particularly his *L'évolutionnisme des idées-forces* of 1890, were well known in Spain at the end of the nineteenth century. Fouillée's ideas were disseminated in Spain through the essays of Clarín and Adolfo Posada's *Ideas pedagógicas modernas* of 1892 (Olmedo Moreno 82). Ganivet himself cites Fouillée during his dis-

---

[10] Paradoxically, the center of this territorial character of Spain is Castile and not Andalucía, where both Ganivet and Seneca were born. In Ganivet's rewriting of Spain's history the birth-place of Seneca does not fit in with the development of Castilian hegemony. If Seneca can be mythologized into a national political figure then his origin can be accordingly adjusted: "que a nacer más tarde, en la Edad Media, quizá no naciera en Andalucía, sino en Castilla."

cussion of aboulia in the *Idearium español,* and Ganivet's concept of "fuerzas madres" closely approximates Fouillée's notion of "idées forces."

The notion of "idées forces" corresponded to the vitality Fouillée ascribed to the psychologic aspect of the human organism at both the individual and social level. In this sense they can be understood as a reservoir of what is commonly called "will-power." The role of the "idées forces" was not held to be the passive representation of exterior causes, but rather the active intervention of internal mental energy in the process of evolution, a theory which Fouillée offered as a corrective to the exclusive agency Darwin assigned to natural selection: "Darwin n'a pas assez considéré les nécessités intérieures, soit physiologiques, soit psychologiques, qui agissent avant toute sélection et rendent la sélection même possible" (1: 78).

For this reason the proper cultivation and conservation of the energy engendered by this force was considered crucial to any society or nation which sought to develop in harmony with its "natural" territorial and racial character. As Olmedo Moreno has pointed out, Fouillée's introduction of relatively independent psychic factors contradicts the greater naturalist determinism of his thought. This contradiction is played out in the *Idearium español,* where the indiscriminate squandering of the "idées-forces" debilitates the underlying territorial spirit. That which is supposedly transcendental and eternal in the national physiognomy is subject to the historically grounded conditions in which ideas become manifest in the individual or collective psyche. For Ganivet ideas may come out of territorial or purely idealist formations, but they are also affected by the specific psychological energy which gives them form, an energy which is intersected by other psycho-biological concerns. In this way ideas are dependent upon psychic states for their energy and realization; or, as Olmedo Moreno states, ideas must:

> buscar la fuente de esa energía en los estados más cargados de tensión, sea *deseo* o *aversión*, es decir, en los de placer o dolor, incluso en los estados cenestésicos, que por su continuidad, parecen poseer más la permanencia que requiere la energía. Así el valor de las ideas como modeladoras de la acción resulta más bien relativo a los movimientos de *apetencia* o *repulsión* que provocan, con lo que se oscurece su objetividad y su validez transubjetiva. (my italics 85)

Olmedo-Moreno alludes to a point that I would like to elaborate further. The binary tensions and movements of desire and repulsion which Fouillée (and subsequently Ganivet) viewed as the main source for the energy and subsistence of ideas are certainly not timeless constructs of the human mind or psyche. As I have argued, they are the conceptual and discursive products of the nineteenth century's neurological and psychological channeling of notions, discourses and practices surrounding sexuality, gender and physical vitality.

Significantly, Ganivet refers to this psychic energy as a "fuerza madre," a de-sexualized gendering of the ideal whose basis in the negation of female sexuality-subjectivity becomes clearer in the light of his preoccupation with virgin-birth. For Ganivet and the male imagination of the turn-of-the-century, the feminine is the low, the other, the mass, the corporal, the sexually degenerative threat to the masculine self of high culture. Yet while this ideal energy is defined in terms which deny and subordinate the female, it is simultaneously defined in the terms of a chaste and conserved male potency. Ganivet's Seneca expresses the masculine refusal to be subordinated, drained and deflated by female sexuality. The virility of the masculine ideal is preserved, nothing flows away. This potency is affirmed as a symbolic phallus, the "high" which differentiates the male and the masculine ideal from the "low" of femininity and material reality: "mantente de tal modo *firme* y *erguido*, que al menos se pueda decir de ti que eres un hombre" (my italics). The threat to this masculine ideal energy is dissolution through sexual contact with women or men or masturbation. Ganivet warns against this degeneration encoding it within a co-functional opposition which contrasts the exterior, "nada extraño a tu espíritu" and the interior, "tienes dentro de ti." The interior is the sexually energized yet chaste masculine ideal while the exterior is feminine socio-sexual corruption, the libidinal coding for liberal democracy and capitalism, which will "envilecernos con su contacto."

Ganivet's appropriation of Seneca combines anxiety about sexuality with the objective authority of medical science. Through Seneca Ganivet introduces his theory of psychic-national debilitation in the reciprocal discourses of nineteenth-century sexology and medicine. In this sense it is important to note that Ganivet not only extols Seneca as a true Spanish philosopher, but also as a doctor or *sangrador* who "ha influido en nuestras ciencias médicas tanto como Hipócrates o Galeno" (47).

In the discursive fusion of the period sexuality itself is silenced or displaced to a discourse opposing the "normal" to the "pathological." Sexual behaviors, later to be assigned to sexual "identities," were mediated through clinical discussions of nervous disorders, masturbation and other forms of non-reproductive "excess."[11] The *Idearium español* borrows from this discourse of medicalized sexuality, conceiving of the nation as a sufferer of a kind of "pathological abatement." This application of a clinical model to the nation presupposes that the nation itself could be analyzed with the same methodologies and instruments as an individual patient. The nation is conceived as a unified, organic body whose reserves and flows of vital sexual energy become synonymous with internal and foreign policy:

> El individuo, a su vez, es una reducción fotográfica de la sociedad: la vida individual fisiológica es una combinación de la energía vital interna con las fuerzas exteriores absorbidas y asimiladas; la vida espiritual se desarrolla de un modo análogo, nutriéndose el espíritu de los elementos ideales que la sociedad conserva como almacenados, según la expresión de Fouillée. En este sentido, creo yo que es provechosa la aplicación de la psicología individual a los estados sociales, y la patología del espíritu a la patología política. (164)

Thus Ganivet's aim in the *Idearium español* is to follow the gradual and long-term dissipation of Spain's "energía vital interna" in order to determine whether its sexual-historical excess has been in keeping with its independent territorial spirit. Beginning with the Reconquest, Spain started out with a full reservoir of vital energy amassed during a saintly cause: "La energía acumulada en nuestra lucha contra los árabes no era sólo energía guerrera, como muchos creen; era según haré ver después, energía espiritual" (107). For Ganivet the long period of the Reconquest was a time when the

---

[11] Foucault has described this medicalization of sexuality in *The History of Sexuality:* "This was in fact a science made up of evasions since, given its inability or refusal to speak of sex itself, it concerned itself primarily with aberrations, perversions, exceptional oddities, pathological abatements, and morbid aggravations." (53)

masculine solidarity and chastity of the warrior spirit was united against the feminine sensuality of the Arabs. The spiritually and historically logical course of action would have been to pursue the struggle into Africa but, as Ganivet laments, the "discovery" of America and European intrigue led Spain elsewhere. A young and immature nation spends its precious and limited energies in the New World and the Low Countries:

> apenas constituida la nación, nuestro espíritu se sale del cauce que le estaba marcado y se derrama por todo el mundo en busca de glorias exteriores y vanas, quedando la nación convertida en un cuartel de reserva, en un hospital de inválidos, en un semillero de mendigos. (105)

In the discourse of nineteenth-century psychology, Spain, an immature and developing youth, forgoes the righteous path of chaste maturation, here analogous to the spiritual-national pursuit of the Reconquest into Africa, and enters into premature and debilitating sexual relations or colonial expansion in Europe and the New World which "atraía y seducía como cosa de encantamiento" (75). [12] Spain's vital energies are literally and indiscriminately "spilled" ("se derrama") all over the world through colonization, making the nation into a hospital or breeding ground ("semillero") for the clinically or economically exhausted, who are "debilitados por un gasto incesante de energía" (116).

This image of Spain as a sickly youth, particularly the notion that Spain had "spilled" its energies, borrows from the contemporary literature warning against the ravaging effects of "non-conceptive" sexual acts, be they the result of contraception, homosexual activity or masturbation. All such acts threatened manliness, virtue and the nation as personified by Seneca in the *Idearium español*. As early as 1760 André Tissot, in his treatise *L'Onanisme*, gave a medical rewriting to religious injunctions against non-conceptive sex, cautioning that masturbatory excess sapped the soul's spiritual strength (Mosse 28). Tissot and later nineteenth-century sexologists

---

[12] When reading Ganivet's pieties about the righteous "spiritual expansion" into Northern Africa that should have followed the Reconquest, it is important to recall Spain's ongoing commercial interest and colonial intervention in Morocco in the late nineteenth and early twentieth centuries which had none of the moral tone he spoke of.

felt that sexual excess physically and mentally debilitated the individual, leaving him or her weak and indecisive, symptoms akin to Ganivet's usage of the concept of aboulia. The renowned nineteenth century sexologist Richard von Krafft-Ebing solidified the connection between sexual excess, nervous disorders and national degeneration in his *Psychopathia sexualis* of 1877, linking sexual excess with modernization and urbanization.

GANIVET AS DOCTOR: NATURAL HISTORY AS NATIONAL HISTORY

Ganivet's discussion of Spain's spiritual and material circumstances is, in other words, clearly grounded in medical terms which conflate theories of sexual activity and mental-physical morbidity with foreign and domestic policies which over-stimulate and weaken the nation. Since Ganivet believes, in accord with the organicist model, that the nation's fortunes can be compared to individual health or pathology, he employs the instruments and theories of medical and psychological science in the *Idearium español*. The text situates the rhetoric of politics within the model of clinical discourse, empowering itself through the socially determined "objectivity" and authority invested in the medical disciplines. In this instance Ganivet assumes the clear-headed, critical distance from his subject that a doctor does from a patient. It is a disguise which authorizes, legitimizes and sanctifies his analysis and more importantly, perhaps, his personal investment in the same. In the final section of the *Idearium español* Ganivet makes clear the discursive authority he has assumed from the outset: "Si yo fuese consultado como médico espiritual para formular el diagnóstico del padecimiento que los españoles sufrimos..." (162). Here Ganivet attempts to gain the authority ascribed to a doctor when one verbally seeks their assistance, a request which implicitly recognizes wisdom and authority. Yet obviously he was not in fact *consultado* as a "spiritual doctor" nor as any other kind of practitioner. His authority, diagnosis and cure are unsolicited. In the same passage Ganivet goes on to back his own assumed scientific authority with that of well-known psychologist-neurologists of the period: "y la sostendría, si necesario fuera, con textos de autoridades y examen de casos clínicos muy detallados, pues desde Esquirol y Maudsley hasta Ribot y Pierre Janet hay una larga serie de médicos y psicólogos que han estudiado esta enfermedad,..." [13] Yet, as Ricardo Senabre has convincingly demonstrated, the only authority among these for which Ganivet could claim a first-hand reading knowledge was Ribot, whose *Les maladies de la volonté* contained detailed references to the degeneracy theorists Ganivet cited (597).

Grounding medical authority within the national tradition, Ganivet makes a passing reference to the sixteenth-century Spanish biologist-theologian Miguel Serveto, a pioneer in pulmonary circulation. As with the reference to Seneca noted before, Ganivet seeks to locate himself within a tradition of Spanish spiritual healers of his own creation:

> la interminable falange de sangradores impertérritos, que durante siglos se han encargado de aligerar el aparato circulatorio de los españoles, enviando a muchos a la fosa, es cierto, pero purgando a los demás de sus excesos sanguíneos a fin de que pudiesen vivir en relativa paz y calma. (48)

This hyperbolic, heroic narrative of intrepid Spanish bloodletters who kill as many patients as they help would be little more than an enigmatic or comic absurdity if we do not discern the underlying motives and functions of its metaphors. As in the case of the Virgin wherein Ganivet creates a paradigm for spiritual purity, the reference to bloodletters, particularly the emphasis on circulation, seeks to create a mythology of national healers dedicated to the circulation or regeneration of national vitality. As with the discourse of sexual debilitation, the notion of controlling or eliminating "excesos" is crucial to the project of national renovation. But unlike the discourse of sexual debilitation, whose basis is the retention of vitality and *fluids*, the circulatory model associates conservation with "old" or degenerate blood in need of purging.

The historically immediate and influential predecessor for Ganivet's equating the historian with the doctor is Hippolyte Taine. [14] Taine was greatly influenced by the inter-related national

---

[13] Here Ganivet is referring, in chronological order, to important theorist-practitioners of degeneracy theory: Jean-Etienne Esquirol, *Des maladies mentales* (1838); Henry Maudsley, *The Physiology and Pathology of Mind* (1867); Théodule Ribot, *L'hérédité psychologique* (1873) and *Les maladies de la volonté* (1887); Pierre Janet, *Etat mental des hystériques; les accidents mentaux* (1894).

[14] I am indebted to H. Ramsden's "Similarities in Taine" from his book *The 1898 Movement in Spain* (51-64), for my discussion of Taine's influence on Ganivet.

disasters of 1870-71, the Franco-Prussian war and the Commune, which led him to view contemporary French history as an illness dating back to the social transformations brought about by the Revolution of 1789. As Ganivet in the *Idearium español*, Taine viewed the crisis of France as a psychological problem and applied the principles of individual psychology to the nation. Taine himself made this quite clear in his well-known statement that "je n'ai jamais fait que de la psychologie appliquée ou la psychologie pure, chacune des deux aidant l'autre" (Ramsden, *1898 Movement* 52). In his *Histoire de la littérature anglaise*, Taine refers to himself as "un médecin consultant" (Ramsden, *1898 Movement* 52), a striking similarity to, and perhaps the actual origin of the *Idearium español*'s "si yo fuese consultado como médico..." Taine felt that only through giving politics and politicians a basis in biological science could the nation's ills be diagnosed and cured. His writings sought to provide this formation: "mon livre sera une consultation de médecins," "un mémoire à consulter par les hommes qui sont ou qui peuvent devenir des hommes d'Etat" (Ramsden, *1898 Movement* 53). Taine thus proposes that Machiavelli's Prince go to medical school. Consequently, for Taine, Ganivet and others influenced by Taine's historical writings, the nation is conceptualized in a binarism of health-illness, an opposition that could also be stated in terms of tradition-transformation. The conception of the nation is conflated with the medical opposition of the sick and the healthy, an alliance that encodes specific partisan socio-political programs within a biologically positive or negative scale of value. In order to diagnose the illness or social transformations afflicting the nation and to prescribe a cure compatible with its physical-spiritual constitution, a project of self-knowledge, of defining the natural, healthy and eternal essence of the people or nation is required.

This urgent need for self-knowledge is at once personal and collective in the *Idearium español*. It is personal in two ways: first in that the model for this introspection is the psychological study of the individual; secondly because Ganivet takes this model to heart, directly and indirectly offering himself as a case study of the national problem. Individual psychological-spiritual introspection is projected onto the nation in the guise of an isolationist proposal, one that will allow Spain to turn inward in an act of self-consciousness and self-preservation. Speaking as a doctor, specifically a psy-

chologist, Ganivet sets out the practical and theoretical traps of
psychological study. His cautionary remarks are grounded in the
binarism interior-exterior which, as we have seen, is so basic to the
text: "El problema más difícil de resolver en el estudio psicológico,
en el que han encallado los investigadores más perspicuos, es el de
enlazar con rigor lógico la experiencia interna con los fenómenos
exteriores" (65). What follows can only be characterized as an ironic warning against psychologists who construct "dangerous ideologies" based on the theoretical abstraction and universalization of
tendencies they find in themselves. To the reader who is familiar
with Ganivet's life, habits and correspondence, this statement and
the ensuing discussion of "misanthropes," "ascetics," and men who
are "apto para vivir en la celda de un convento" can only be an expression of self-criticism or parody. Aside from the problem of an-
alytical self-projection on the part of the psychologist, the conceptual importance of this review of the potential pitfalls of individual
analysis is its critique of superficial exterior manifestations and its
sense of the necessity to discover the secret, internal workings of
individual consciousness. Ganivet compares two superficially similar ascetic figures, Kempis and Fray Luis de Granada, differentiating and qualifying their internal paths to asceticism. He characterizes Kempis' asceticism as an abstract ontology which reflects "un
alma enfermiza linfática," whereas Fray Luis de Granada is said to
arrive at asceticism through his profound knowledge and contact
with reality and humanity, indicating a healthy "alma robusta, san-
guínea."

   At this point in the text there is a double shift from individual
to national psychology and from a psychological to an evolutionist
and determinist model. Linking the psychological to the determinist approach is the overriding concern to overcome the empirical
and interpretative limitations of studying the "exterior" phenomena
of national or natural history. For Ganivet, nearly all of Spain's real
social, economic and political history since the time of the Reconquest, up to and including the modernization and socio-economic
transformation of the turn-of-the-century, constituted "exterior"
experience. According to this argument the exterior history of
Spain is a series of accidents, mistakes and lost opportunities based
on the misinterpretation of the national spirit. What Ganivet seeks
to uncover in the *Idearium español* is the hidden and eternal interi-
or psychology or essence of the nation:

> De igual modo, cuando se estudia la estructura psicológica de un país, no basta representar el mecanismo externo, ni es prudente explicarlo mediante una ideología fantástica: hay que ir más hondo y buscar en la realidad misma el núcleo irreductible al que están adheridas todas las envueltas que van transformando en el tiempo la fisionomía de este país. Y como siempre que se profundiza se va a dar en lo único que hay para nosotros perenne, la tierra, ese núcleo se encuentra en el "espíritu territorial." (66)

In this brief passage Ganivet changes from a psychologist to a philosopher of natural science, attributing the evolution of national psychology to the hidden forces of geography. Ganivet claims that specific geographic formations have a particular natural personality which they impart to the peoples who inhabit them. Briefly stated, island nations are said to be aggressive, continental nations are patriotic and peninsular nations are independent. These arbitrary and supposedly universal territorial personalities are based on a selective review of the nineteenth-century histories of England, France and Spain respectively, three historically competitive imperial rivals. That these nations themselves or many other examples throughout the world contradict this geographical thesis is dismissed as instances of a lack of self-knowledge, misinterpretation or the incomplete evolution of the territorial ideal. It is precisely this gap between the hidden, eternal interior and the superficial, transitory exterior which preoccupies Ganivet in the *Idearium español*, a contradiction he seeks to investigate through critical juxtaposition: "La evolución de España se explica sólo cuando se contrastan todos los hechos exteriores de su historia con el espíritu permanente, invariable, que el territorio crea, infunde, mantiene en nosotros" (67).

This statement is yet another reiteration of the text's introductory simile contrasting the ephemeral, exterior sensuality of material history with the permanent, internal experience of spiritual virginity. This initial contrast situates Spanish history in a violent parable of forced maternity, namely rape, wherein Spain is at once the victim and the perpetrator. Consequently, the evolution of the territorial spirit and the external socio-political history which violates it is narrated in an ambiguous, sympathetic and unsympathetic logic of self-blame. The territorial drive towards independence at all costs is blamed for the lack of self-knowledge and the ensuing divisive and self-destructive behavior.

It is also necessary to ground the psycho-sexual dynamics of Ganivet's geographical determinism in the political atmosphere of late nineteenth-century Spain. Ganivet's insistence upon an eternal, unified national spirit centered in Castile must be read in the light of the emergence of strong nationalist movements in Catalonia and the Basque provinces. These historical developments, according to Ganivet, constituted a divergence from the unified Castilian essence of the nation (Labanyi 132). As Joe Labanyi has pointed out, the rural backwardness of Castile contrasted with the industrial economies of the competing nationalist regions (133). This lent Castile a timeless, traditional anchoring in the face of modernity in the same way that the chaste and traditionally grounded figures of the Virgin and Seneca functioned as images of an immutable national essence. Ganivet enabled himself to dismiss history and these contemporary political challenges by assigning an ahistorical, geographically determined love of independence to the national character.

At times the idea of strong-willed independence is grounded in the familiar discourse of restrained or unrestrained sexuality. In this instance the text makes an association between independence and promiscuity, an association which places the responsibility for the sexual, spiritual and historical rape of the national symbol (the Virgin) on the Spanish people itself. Thus, in that gray area between symbols and national allegories, the Virgin and the nation are held responsible for their own victimization:

> ...somos una "casa con dos puertas", y por lo tanto, "mala de guardar", y como nuestro partido constante fue dejarlas abiertas, por temor que las fuerzas dedicadas a vigilarlas se volviesen contra nosotros mismos, nuestro país se convirtió en una especie de parque internacional, donde todos los pueblos y razas han venido a distraerse cuando les ha parecido oportuno; nuestra historia es una serie inacabable de invasiones y de expulsiones, una guerra permanente de independencia. (71)

Here Ganivet employs a euphemistic and domestic terminology of chastity and promiscuity to describe foreign intervention and ethnic diversity in Spain. Spain, previously figured as a virgin is now colloquially configured as a poorly defended "house" with two "doors" or openings. Ganivet then shifts to biological and sensual terms in

his description of the various "peoples and races" who have entered
through these wantonly accessible architectural orifices in order to
"amuse themselves" whenever they felt like it. Instead of a virgin,
Spain is a "parque internacional," an open-house, a whore.

Compounding the difficulties presented by the uncooperative
peninsular spirit, Ganivet claims that Spain's mountainous geographical barriers have exacerbated its independent spirit, giving
the nation the additional and misguided aggressiveness of an island-
nation: "En realidad nos hemos creído insulares, y quizá este error
explique muchas anomalías de nuestra historia" (71). This combination of extreme independence and aggressiveness has distorted
and debilitated the national spirit in a way which is co-functional to
the sexual-political squandering of the nation's stoic and virginal
energies. This link is most obvious in the case of Spain's colonial
enterprise in the Americas. It is less obvious in Ganivet's surrepti-
tious allusions to the divisive Catalan and Basque separatist movements of turn-of-the-century Spain.

What Ganivet describes in sexual-"medical" terms as the wast-
ing or *spilling* of the nation's vital energies in the New World was
motivated by the desire to finance radical independence movements in the peninsula: "y como la preponderancia futura de Castilla era un amago contra la independencia de los demás, nació
espontáneamente, como eflorescencia de nuestro espíritu territorial,
la idea de buscar fuera del suelo español fuerzas para ser indepen-
dientes en España" (73). For Ganivet the failure to discern and act
in accordance with the independent territorial spirit in the best interests of the nation, what he calls a lack of "sentido sintético," or "la
facultad de apreciar en su totalidad nuestros varios intereses políti-
cos," has resulted in the prolonged Arab occupation, the political
partition of the peninsula, the catastrophe of the Armada, nationally debilitating colonization in Europe and the New World, the loss
of Gibraltar, a dysfunctional court system and incessant civil and regional strife. In the arts and literature the independent national
character has produced a body of work of very irregular and undisciplined quality. Instead of aesthetic schools or literary movements
Spanish arts and letters have been characterized by strongly indi-
vidualistic expressions of genius or failure. The achievements of
such luminaries as Velázquez, Goya, Calderón and Cervantes, although laudable in themselves, did not lead to the development of
universal trends. Importantly, Ganivet views this self-inhibiting in-

dependence in a fatalist and somewhat dispassionate light. For him this is the inexorable evolution of the territorial spirit: "¿Es imposible en absoluto modificar estos instintos de insubordinación que nos destrozan y nos aniquilan? Yo creo que no" (104).

The question arises whether Ganivet's theory of geographical determinism constitutes a naturalist or positivist doctrine. Given Ganivet's idealist if not platonic conception of ideas, aesthetics, matter and the body, a materially and literally grounded (in land) conception of human character or history seems contradictory. To better understand this contradiction it is once again necessary to study the influence of Taine on Ganivet. Taine himself is often considered to be a prime example of nineteenth-century naturalism, but as both H. Ramsden and Guillermo Díaz-Plaja have observed, Taine's determinism has decidedly metaphysical underpinnings. Taine sought to abstract universal laws from facts and saw little value in the facts themselves. In this sense science merely serves the aesthetic-metaphysical search for universal ideals. As Ramsden has pointed out, Taine saw his thought as a compromise between the English emphasis on empiricism and the German privileging of abstraction (*1898 Movement* 66). The subservience of facts to universal laws empowers interpretation over empirical study. It was this complementary relationship between empiricism and Hegelian universals that led Taine to the natural scientists who framed universal laws from their study of specific organisms. Specific events or periods of history could be studied and recorded, but according to Taine such empirical observation is only productive if it aides in the uncovering and interpretation of underlying psychological laws. Here, psychology is synonymous with universal and eternal essence. It is at this point that Taine's thought, as well as that of those he influenced in the Generation of '98, becomes acutely ambiguous.

The interchangeable equation of territorial-national essence with a territorial-national psychology ascribes, *a priori*, a fundamentally arbitrary and metaphysical interpretation to the "scientific" discipline of psychology. In this instance the historian, in a partisan response to specific historical developments, undertakes the contemporary discursive and conceptual necessity of "science" in order to support older ideological, moral and philosophical positions against liberal democracy and industrialization. The empirically observable socio-historical components of psychology, namely the ways in which socio-economic, political and even technical transformations affect our public and intimate psyche are ignored in favor of a metaphysical faith in the hermeneutic of territorial determinism.

In the *Idearium español* Ganivet surpasses Taine's ambiguity concerning the sciences and assumes a strikingly anti-positivist position. His principal criticism centers around the notion of a purely practical and empirical basis for knowledge independent of metaphysical or hermeneutic absolutes. Scientific method and materialism had disrupted the connection between reason and the faith in underlying, transcendental forces (religion or geographical determinism): "El criticismo ha desligado la razón de la fe, el positivismo ha querido desligar el conocimiento de la razón, el materialismo ha intentado destruir la base misma del conocimiento" (56). Furthermore, for Ganivet the practical and empirical sciences, which he qualified in bodily and perhaps biblically satirical terms as "'nuevos órganos' de conocimiento," are associated with the vulgar and corporeal realism of the external world, the body and their socio-economic and biological reproduction while the metaphysical ideal remains eternally and hygienically pure. His biting critique of positivism does not, however, rule out his appropriation of the lexicon of evolution, degeneration, geographical determinism and psychology in order to theoretically modernize his anti-modernist idealism. Although there are few passages in the *Idearium español* which vigorously or extensively apply evolutionary or biological theories, there are superficial aesthetic and philosophical appropriations of these discourses which lend an air of "scientific" objectivity to the text as in the following anatomical imagery:

> La síntesis espiritual de un país es su arte. Pudiera decirse que el espíritu territorial es la medula; la religión, el cerebro; el espíritu guerrero, el corazón; el espíritu jurídico, la musculatura, y el espíritu artístico, como una red nerviosa que todo lo enlaza y lo mueve. (96)

As we have already seen in the case of the medicalization of sexuality and the stoic discourse of the preservation of sexual-national energies, Ganivet is quite adept at lending a modern, scientific tone to his basically anti-modern ideology. At times Ganivet will employ a positivist argument only to subsequently qualify and debunk it in the same passage. Immediately after attributing the specific development of ideas in Spain to its particular climate and race: "por ser diferente nuestro clima y nuestra raza," a typically positivist logic, he goes on to challenge the utility of science in Spain: "A la vista está nuestro desvío de las ciencias de aplicación: no hay medio de hacerlas arraigar en España,..." And in yet another of those moments which resound with innocent self-critique, Ganivet would seem to describe his own personal application of science: "Y no es que no haya hombres de ciencia, los ha habido y los hay, pero cuando no son de inteligencia mediocre, se sienten arrastrados hacia las alturas donde la ciencia se desnaturaliza, combinándose ya con la religión, ya con el arte" (98). Although Ganivet may not view himself primarily as a "scientist," this self-appointed doctor does employ the terminologies of psychological, neurological and determinist science to substantiate his own moral-philosophical or ideological positions.

COLONIALISM AND DEGENERATION: THE STORY OF AGATÓN TINOCO

The explicit political recommendation of the *Idearium español* calls for national introspection, isolation and withdrawal. Yet while the text does indeed champion the need for a contemplative, inward, spiritual regeneration, this fact does not preclude the coexistence and co-functioning of other transnational political and cultural agendas. In fact Ganivet's call for national renewal reflects an intellectual-cultural will to power in the former and contemporary colonies. The discursively out of place tale of Agatón Tinoco, which Ganivet knowingly qualifies as "un suceso vulgarísimo," serves as an illustrative, if not homey parable of Spain's ongoing role in the future of Latin America. Before entering into an analysis of this autobiographical anecdote, it is necessary to briefly review other passages which address the ties between Spain and Spanish America.

A central concern of Ganivet in the *Idearium español* is the recuperation of Spanish influence in the former and contemporarily rebelling colonies. This concern is premised upon a theoretical differentiation between Spanish and Anglo-Saxon or continental European colonization. This theoretization situates a revisionist or apologist view of history within the contemporary polemic surrounding the alleged socio-biological degeneracy of the Americas. For Ganivet, the non-Hispanic colonization of the Americas and

Africa was born of the drive for independence, security and national consolidation that the material and territorial scarcity of the colonizing nations did not provide. This political impetus quickly became economic, and for Ganivet, ignoble: "su colonización se transformó en negocio útil, práctico, sin duda, pero que ya no era tan noble..." (79) Lacking any profound spiritual or moral motives for their colonization, nations such as Holland and primarily England, were unable to infuse their colonies with the mark of their territorial personalities. According to this vision, non-Spanish economic colonization constituted a failure of national-spiritual insemination, or worse, as in the case of the Belgian Congo, economically motivated genocide. Whereas Ganivet's discussion of European colonization offers insightful elements for an analysis of the role of colonization in the formation of national European states as well as the development of mercantilism, his analysis of Spanish conquest and colonialism in the Americas is decidedly less materialist. He denounces the literature of the "Black Legend" and refers to the conquistadors as "legítimos guerrilleros" who conquered not out of greed, but out of a misdirected build-up of chaste, spiritual, warrior energy accumulated during the Reconquest of Spain. According to Ganivet, North Africa would have been the logical site for the organic continuation of the Reconquest. Instead, this morally "pure" energy was transmitted to the Americas, the violent and sexual means of which is not mentioned, imprinting Spain's geographically determined independent spirit in the colonies. This belligerently independent spirit mixed with the local colonial territorial personalities giving birth to new configurations. For Ganivet it is this youth which accounts for the ongoing civil strife and material poverty in Latin America. Importantly, Ganivet interprets this conflict as a sign of *health* and not a symptom of European degeneration in the New World as did many of his contemporaries in both Spain and Latin America. Unlike the United States, which Ganivet felt had artificially assumed the superficial political and economic structures of its geographically evolved colonizer, Latin America had organically reverted to the initial stage of a new social configuration like a healthy new-born child. In this way Ganivet reiterated Hegel's notion that Latin America was spiritually immature. Yet as did his Uruguayan contemporary Rodó, Ganivet sought to minimize the negative connotations that the German philosopher had also associated with Latin America's youth, as in the following passage from the *Idearium español*:

Las naciones hispanoamericanas no han pasado de la infancia, en tanto que los Estados Unidos han comenzado por la edad viril. ¿Por qué? Porque las unas, al recibir la influencia de sus territorios, han retrocedido y han comenzado la evolución como pueblos jóvenes, paso a paso, tropezando en los escollos en que tropiezan las sociedades nuevas que carecen de un exacto conocimiento del camino que deben seguir; y la otra ha continuado viviendo una vida artificial, importada de Europa, como pudiera vivir en cualquier territorio, por ejemplo, en Australia. (128)

What is interesting in this passage is the way in which it simultaneously employs and criticizes the complementary discourses of evolution and degeneration. In loosely associated biological, sociological and spiritual terminology Ganivet defines Latin American societies as telluric hybrids which have regressed to an initial stage of a loosely defined idealist evolution. Yet he is quick to differentiate his conceptual usage of the discourses of evolution and regression from the allied discourse of biological degeneration. What other commentators viewed as social instability, conflict or biological inferiority Ganivet saw as the potential for a superior evolution or what he calls in the *Idearium español*: "la promesa de una futura superioridad de nuestra raza." Evidently, as his usage of the possessive adjective *nuestra* demonstrates, Ganivet does not distinguish between the Spanish and Spanish American "race(s)." Despite his assertions of a purely spiritual interest in preserving the bonds of cultural and racial fraternity: "la vecindad, la conciudadanía, la raza, el idioma, la religión, la historia, la comunidad de intereses o de cultura," his construction of the post-colonial relationship retains the paternalism and possessiveness of the unequal colonial relationship. Moreover, for Ganivet to speak of post-colonial reconciliation while Spain was actively maintaining severely repressive colonial administrations in Cuba and Puerto Rico, is to engage in idealist, political sophistry. It is precisely his white-washed and immaterial version of the original colonial structures that Ganivet wishes to re-establish: "Si España quiere recuperar su puesto, ha de esforzarse para restablecer su propio prestigio intelectual, y luego para llevarlo a América e implantarlo sin aspiraciones utilitarias" (132).

In this way Spain could return to Latin America as a mature and materially disinterested parent to give socio-cultural guidance to these youthful nations, an idea not at all unlike the original ideology of "civilizing the savages" promoted by contemporary apologists of the conquest. In the *Idearium español* Ganivet himself lives out this political fantasy in his personal anecdote about Agatón Tinoco, a tale which he says will show that his ideas are not just "palabrería," but that they have "un sentido muy justo y muy práctico." As Ganivet tells us, while working as a consul in Antwerp he was brought to the hospital to comfort "un español, que deseaba hablar con la autoridad de su país" as he lay dying from "fiebre amarilla o africana" contracted as a colonist in the Belgian Congo. Functioning simultaneously as a priest and as a socially recognized as well as fictionally self-constructed national authority, Ganivet listens to the confession of the suffering colonist. Importantly, the first utterance of Tinoco's directly recorded by Ganivet was his apologetic confession "Yo no soy español..." Ganivet reassures Tinoco that the hospital's mistake was logical in that although Tinoco may not be Spanish, "lo parece." Tinoco rejoins once again that he is not Spanish, specifying his origin: "Yo soy de Centroamérica, señor, de Managua, y mi familia era portuguesa; me llamo Agatón Tinoco." At this point Ganivet authoritatively (and consciously) cuts off the confession to deny what has just been said and to didactically correct Tinoco with the following assertion: "Entonces – interrumpí yo –, es usted español por tres veces." Up to this point Ganivet's account of the meeting depicts a discursive struggle over the identity of Tinoco: the hospital assumed he was Spanish but Tinoco denies it; Ganivet says that he looks and sounds like a Spaniard but Tinoco differentiates himself in terms of region, nation and colonial-familial origin. In one sentence Ganivet negates these three points of difference, re-establishing paternity and, more importantly, reasserting the national unity and authority of Spain (and himself as its authorized representative) despite Iberian and colonial rifts.

Tinoco's life-story is one of heroic misfortune: he fled his home to save face after conjugal infidelity, labored in one of the unsuccessful attempts to build the Panama canal and finally went to the Congo as a colonist and contracted a fatal disease. After listening to Tinoco, Ganivet delivers a sermon on his life that praises Tinoco for his silent martyrdom of epochal and selfless toil. The last rites which Ganivet administers in this recreated dialogue repeat the notion of the misguided, self-less and heroic deeds described earlier in

his discussion of the conquistadors. Whereas the conquest and colonization of the Americas constitute the noble yet territorially discordant source of national debilitation and illness, for Tinoco the
neo-imperialist projects of the Panama Canal and African colonization have been the origin of Tinoco's illness. Echoing sentiments
voiced in his description of the materially disinterested but spiritually passionate conquistadors, Ganivet says of Tinoco that his endeavor "ha sido noblísima, puesto que no sólo ha trabajado para
vivir, sino que ha acudido como soldado de fila a prestar su concur-
so a empresas gigantescas..." Continuing his parable of Spain
through the story of Tinoco Ganivet says that he comes from:

> una raza de luchadores y de triunfadores, postrada hoy y humi-
> llada por propias culpas, entre las cuales no es la menor la falta
> de espíritu fraternal, la desunión, que nos lleva a ser juguete de
> poderes extraños y a muchos como usted anden rodando por el
> mundo, trabajando como oscuros peones cuando pudieran ser
> amos con holgura. (136)

Here Ganivet is repeating his thesis that the origin of Spain's trou-
bles, of its illness, lies in its own divisive independent spirit which
leads it into grandiose projects of displaced self-fulfillment and illness. A specific grammatical link between Tinoco's illness and
Spain's national debilitation is the shift away from third person sin-
gular parts of speech ("usted," "le," "su") positing Tinoco as the
exclusive referent to the first person plural direct object pronoun
nos ("que *nos* lleva a ser juguete"). Instead of being the exclusive
subject and addressee of Ganivet's sermon, Tinoco becomes an ill-
fated and illustrative manifestation of a greater "we."

There is a sinister side to this dialogue between Tinoco and
Ganivet if we consider Tinoco's need to meet with a Spanish-speak-
er who could understand, and importantly, sympathize with his
plight. Tinoco announces his narrative plan to convince Ganivet of
the injustice of his suffering early in their conversation: "Yo soy
muy desgraciado, señor, como no hay otro hombre en el mundo. Si
yo le contara a usted mi vida, vería usted que no le engaño." Significantly, poverty and a search for masculine "honor" impelled Tinoco
to participate in two large-scale projects of neo-colonialism, the
Panama Canal and the Belgian King Leopold's infamous and ruthless exploitation of the Congo. Tinoco is both a victim and a partic-

ipant in these modern and modernizing projects of exploitation. He is driven out of his own region's neo-colonial poverty to further the mobility and interests of Euro-American imperialism in Africa.

As mentioned previously Ganivet was opposed to the modern projects of practical, "utilitarian" colonialism and he particularly condemned Belgian abuses in the Congo. In fact Ganivet's novel *La conquista del reino de Maya por el último conquistador español, Pío Cid* (1897) is an exhaustive renunciation of supposedly "high-minded" European imperialism in Africa. Thus Tinoco's death from "yellow or *African* fever" is more than just a point of realistic information. It is the culminating self-inflicted tragedy of one of the "oscuros peones" of economic colonialism and an index of European moral illness. Perhaps for this reason the details of Tinoco's woes do not inspire Ganivet with what could conventionally be described as sympathy or empathy. In fact what we observe is a rhetorical distancing from the "vulgar" details of an individual's painful decline to a plane of verbose and abstract idealism which negates the specific *pathos* of Tinoco's life. Ganivet's response to this encounter is characterized by an underlying combination of indifference, arrogance and hostility which reflects both a Spanish will to power in the former Spanish-American colonies and an ambivalent identification-repulsion concerning the impotent or the sick.

This story functions as yet another parable for the decline of Spanish influence and the desire to recuperate the same. In this sense Ganivet, the citizen of a politically weak and "impotent" nation, seeks to distance himself from his own national and personal reflection manifested in the person of Tinoco, the allegorically immature Latin American whom he wishes to reinscribe into his paternal-national authority. Ganivet's injunction to Tinoco that he should not resent his sufferings and that he should be proud of his life-long impotence and failure conceals his own Nietzschean fear of self-identity and the masses. The sublimated aggression of the Spaniard senses the vengeful resentment, that which Nietzsche termed "the conspiracy of suffering," of the colonized or oppressed, a danger Nietzsche had previously stated in terms of pathology: "The *sick* are man's greatest danger; *not* the evil, *not* the beasts of prey. Those who are failures from the start, downtrodden, crushed – it is they, the *weakest,* who must undermine life among men, who call into question and poison most dangerously our trust in life, in man, and in ourselves" (*Genealogy* 122).

ABOULIA: THE NATIONAL AUTOBIOGRAPHICAL DIAGNOSIS

In the final section of the *Idearium español* Ganivet declares that the nation is suffering from the clinically observable psychological illness of aboulia. This diagnosis is the culmination of his earlier obsessions with sexual dissipation, the loss of idea-energies and the debilitating transgression of the territorial spirit. Ganivet states that aboulia is the "extinción o debilitación grave de la voluntad," which is characterized by the "influjo de las perturbaciones mentales sobre las funciones orgánicas" (162). The victim of aboulia suffers from a lack of intellectual will, the inability to concentrate and a spiritual and physical lethargy. Central to Ganivet's notion of aboulia is the idea of the loss or degeneration of energy, "un abatimiento de energía funcional," a debilitation which renders mental associations and concentration difficult. The "vital internal energies," "los elementos ideales que la sociedad conserva como almacenados," as in the chaste and bodily conservative and conserving figures of the Virgin and Seneca, have been squandered in territorially discordant projects of colonialization and immoral, utilitarian programs of commercial modernization. It is not only a lessening of internal vital (sexual) energy which prevents the abulic individual from concentrating or forming a plan of action. The abulic individual is also afflicted by the perturbing and distracting effects of an *idée fixe*, an obsession which interferes in the normal co-functioning of what Ganivet calls the "sociability" of ideas. The obsessive focus on an *idée fixe* produces a peculiar kind of paralysis which Ganivet successively terms an "impulsión arrebatada," "movimientos de impulsión," and a "determinación arrebatada." Ganivet employs a discourse of frustrated desire, fecundity and reproduction to describe this paralytic, abulic state:

> en unos casos, la idea fija, que es la que influye más enérgicamente sobre la voluntad, produce la determinación arrebatada, violenta, que alguien confunde con la del alienado; en otros, la idea abstracta o la idea ya vieja, reproducida por la memoria, engendran el deseo débil, impotente, irrealizable; no existen las ideas más fecundas, las ideas sanas que nacen del estudio reflexivo y de la observación consciente de la realidad. (167)

Here Ganivet contrasts a weak or impotent abulic desire with fertile or healthy ideas. Abulic impotency prevents the sufferer from attaining healthy and sexually reproductive ideas. It is the memory of an old, abstract idea, such as original sin, the purity of the Virgin or the fig-leaf of stoicism which distracts and disturbs. The "idea-fija" which Ganivet refers to is his own obsession with sexuality, its repression and subsequent displacement to an ideal plane. It is an obsession which has been foundational to the text since the opening passage about the dogma of the Immaculate Conception, the abstinent purity of Seneca, the rhetoric of high ideals which are "sin mancha," the concern for the conservation or loss of vital internal energies and the psycho-neurological model of aboulia.

The autobiographical nature of the *idée fixe* which Ganivet the doctor employs in his discussion of aboulia simultaneously situates the author as the patient of his own diagnosis. In fact Ganivet invokes himself and the reader of the text as occasional sufferers of aboulia:

> Hay una forma vulgar de la abulia que todos conocemos y a veces padecemos. ¿A quién no le habrá invadido en alguna ocasión esa perplejidad de espíritu, nacida del quebranto de fuerzas o del aplanamiento consiguiente a una inacción prolongada, en que la voluntad, falta de una idea dominante que la mueva, vacilante entre motivos opuestos que se contrabalancean, o dominada por una idea abstracta, irrealizable, permanece irresoluta, sin saber qué hacer y sin determinarse a hacer nada? (162)

According to Ganivet it is only when this mental paralysis becomes chronic that the diagnosis of clinical aboulia can be made. Readings of Ganivet's personal correspondence suggest that he felt himself to be such a case. In 1893 he wrote: "Cada día, me va siendo más difícil concentrar mis ideas y fijar mi pensamiento sobre un objeto determinado" (*Obras* 2: 811). Anticipating the spatial-corporal metaphor of the high and the low ideals later included in the *Idearium español*, Ganivet stated that he could not sufficiently free himself from vulgar reality: "En tal estado, el espíritu que abandonó la realidad por demasiado baja no puede elevarse a la infinitud por demasiado alta." In a letter from May 19th, 1894 to his friend Navarro Ledesma, Ganivet's personal account of sexual frustration approximates the "deseo débil, impotente, irrealizable" of the *ideal* described in the *Idearium español*. It is an episode which prefigures the ambivalent attraction-repulsion of sexuality along with a sublimated hostility to women operating in the idealist discourse of the *Idearium español*. Describing an instance of physical impotence Ganivet writes:

> mi último devaneo amatorio fue con una flamenca monumentalmente hermosísima..., y sin embargo, toda la historia se quedó en los preliminares, pues en el momento álgido... me reintegré en mis "hábitos" y alcé el vuelo. Este asco de la materia se me ha desarrollado gradualmente. (del Pino 5)

Here Ganivet's account of physical impotence very closely resembles the process of physical-spiritual distraction and weakening caused by the *idée fixe* characteristic of aboulia, an illness which he notes has been qualified as a "delirio de contacto" (165). What is personally described as a physical crisis in "el momento álgido" later becomes the idealist discourse of the "idea fija" in the *Idearium español,* an obsession which "cae de la atonía en la exaltación, en la 'idea fija' que le arrastra a la 'impulsión violenta'" (163). Most importantly for a discussion of the *Idearium español*, this intimate account of sexual impotence and repulsion is described as a "disgust" (*asco*) with the "materia," understood as the "subject" or "matter" at hand. It is this discursive fusion between disgust for the material and the corporal which is consistent in Ganivet's personal and literary writing.

Although Ganivet states in the *Idearium español* that his study of aboulia is based on the objective individual psychological model of "casos clínicos," his own personal experience would seem to be of at least equal importance, or, as Herbert Ramsden has succinctly affirmed: "Spain's alleged illness, then, is clearly Ganivet's own" (*Idearium* 89). Nevertheless, Ganivet's use of the term in the *Idearium español* is not solely attributable to his own self-analysis, rather, it is also the product of his literary appropriation of the ideas expressed by Théodule Ribot in his *Les maladies de la volonté*. Not only was Ganivet influenced by the content of Ribot's consideration of aboulia, but, as Ricardo Senabre has shown, he apparently lifted and "modified" passages from Ribot's text (598).

Yet I am not interested here in seeking an absolute correspondence between a historically inaccessible author and a fixed single meaning for one of his texts, but rather in establishing a relationship between discourses of personal and national constitution.

Throughout his discussion of aboulia Ganivet shifts back and forth between the theoretical elaboration of the concept and its extrapolation to the nation. The application of a model based on the functions-dysfunctions of the mind and body of an individual to the abstract, metaphorical level of national or social health involves problematic theoretical assumptions. The primary assumption implied here is that the nation can be conceived as a single, homogenous mind-body whose health or illness closely resembles the patterns of individual patients. At one level we have the premise that a socially, culturally, ethnically, economically or linguistically constructed collectivity can be ascribed the neurological and physiological properties of the individual. In this sense the social is subsumed under particular concepts concerning the corporal and the psychological. A second level of difficulty involves the socio-cultural diversity of Spain acknowledged by Ganivet in the *Idearium español* which would seem to challenge the notion of a monolithic union of mind-body. Ganivet appears to distance himself from these issues when he seeks to differentiate what he terms a case of "collective aboulia" from directly individual models: "Yo no profeso la sociología metafórica que considera las naciones como organismos tan bien determinados como los individuales" (163). Yet the argument that he goes on to elaborate does not contradict his disclaimed "metaphorical sociology." Ganivet claims that society is the end-product of the "force" of its individuals, be they healthy or sick, vital or impotent. It is the concept of internal force, borrowed from Fouillée, which bridges the gap between the individual and society. This force is made possible by the immaterial and acorporal gestation of the idea which contains a medically therapeutic vitality of its own as described by Ganivet in *El porvenir de España*: "La idea tiene en sí eso que llaman los médicos *vis medicatrix*, fuerza curativa interna, espontánea: herida en combate, presto se cura, y aun gana fuerzas para empeñar otro mayor en el que vence" (237). Vital internal energies are conserved or dissipated in the individual and in society according to the same processes, "de un modo análogo," enabling the "aplicación de la psicología individual a los estados sociales, y la patología del espíritu a la patología política" (164).

In this way Ganivet intermittently breaks from his clinical description of the individual manifestations of aboulia to describe the national symptoms. Similar to the abulic individual, Spain is distracted by obsessive ideas and unable to concentrate, an impasse leading to the provocative and previously discussed paralytic impasse: "Nuestra nación hace ya tiempo que está como distraída en medio del mundo. Nada le interesa, nada le mueve de ordinario; mas de repente una idea se fija, y no pudiendo equilibrarse con otras, produce la impulsión arrebatada" (164). Spain's *idée fixe* centers around questions of national honor and prestige such as the split with Portugal, the British occupation of Gibraltar and the loss of the colonial empire. These are the external concerns on which Spain has wasted her internal energies. According to Ganivet Spain has been untrue to its Senecan nature of chaste, introspective meditation. The betrayal of this inward, ascetic virtue equates individual, as well as national spiritual and physical weakness with excessive, external action: "El origen de nuestra decadencia y actual postración se halla en nuestro exceso de acción, en haber acometido empresas enormemente desproporcionadas con nuestro poder..." (169).

The observation that Ganivet projects his own self-diagnosed "illness" onto the nation has itself been characterized as a "sick" act by modern biographers such as Judith Ginsberg who states that such an inability to differentiate the personal from the national "strongly suggests a pathologically grandiose self-image" (100), and by contemporary *fin de siècle* European critics such as Max Nordau, whose Spanish translator, Nicolás Salmerón, wrote in 1902 that Spain's literary youth was characterized by "la debilidad de espíritu, innata o adquirida, y la ignorancia, la predisponen fatalmente al misticismo; la exageración monstruosa de su "yo", de su amor propio, su imposibilidad de atención, la convierten en egoísta" (Díaz-Plaja 12). Comments such as these pose a dilemma to the Ganivet scholar and reveal the author's success in consolidating the paradigm of illness as a defining term for this period in Spanish letters and history. The definition of the "problem of Spain," one of political instability and weakness, of the socially dislocating impact of developing capitalism and industrialization and of the crumbling of a colonial empire were perceived and recorded by Ganivet and his contemporaries as *symptoms* of a greater underlying *illness*, be it of territory, character or race. Yet while it is possible to investigate the personal and historical origins of the discourse of the pathological there is still something relatively arbitrary in this concept in that it is only one of many possible descriptive paradigms for the same series of events. Nevertheless it is important not to confuse or equate the turn-of-the-century sensations of fatigue, impotence and illness with verifiable historical processes or conditions. What I seek to do here is to investigate the personal and socio-historical reality of these perceptions without substituting them for universal historical truths. H. Ramsden expresses similar sentiments in his book *The 1898 Movement in Spain* when he says in a footnote: "I must emphasize that I am not here concerned with what a modern historian might consider *was* the history of Spain, only with what the authors of *En torno al casticismo* and the *Idearium español* believed was the problem of Spain" (12). Nevertheless the critical literature about this period often assumes the historical universality of the discourse of "illness" or "diagnosis" because as Guillermo Díaz-Plaja has stated: "ciertas enfermedades de espíritu careciesen de definición académica." The literature of sickness is deemed "sick literature" both by turn-of-the-century authors such as Nordau and Bourget and by later twentieth century critics who view the act of diagnosis as a sick act in itself.

Sickness as Virtue and the Critique of Capitalism

Ganivet's preoccupation with "the problem of Spain" in the *Idearium español* was the concern of the majority of committed Spanish intellectuals at the turn-of-the-century. Moreover, as is most obvious in the case of Unamuno's *En torno al casticismo*, Ganivet's psychological and medical approach to Spain's political, economic and social problems was anticipated and followed by other writers. What distinguishes the *Idearium español* from other contemporary national *diagnoses* is its ambivalently dynamic deployment of the metaphor of national illness as both a negative and affirmative instrument for the critique of Spain. Whereas the text certainly does describe the purported ills and character faults of the Spanish people and nation, it simultaneously finds a redemptive quality to these frailties. The contradictory dialectic of illness in the *Idearium español* stems from the text's problematic inversion of the oppositions of illness/health and weakness/strength in a way which challenges the conventional hierarchy of inferior and superior nations based on the criteria of material wealth and political power.

In a structurally coherent way this ambivalence concerning illness is linked to the text's foundational discourses of abstinence
and virginity centered around stoicism and the Immaculate Conception. The principal concepts shared by these two doctrines are
the inter-related notions of virtue and morality. In and of themselves as religious concepts and specifically as employed in the
Idearium español, the authority and value of virtue and morality are
directly tied to an association, albeit negative, with sexuality. In this
way virtue and morality are defined in opposition to sexual activity
yet require the repressed presence of the same in order to be recognized as meritorious. Thus the moral well-being of the individual
becomes synonymous with its *health*, a stoic equation pointed out
by Nietzsche in an aphorism from *The Gay Science*: "*Health of the
Soul.* – The popular medical formulation of morality goes back to
Ariston of Chios, 'virtue is the health of the soul,' would have to
be changed to become useful, at least to read: '*your* virtue is the
health of *your* soul'" (176). In this way the reciprocal moralization
of health and the medicalization of morality contributed to the belief that "excessive" sexual activity debilitated the mind, body and
soul, or, in the case of the *Idearium español*, wasted internal vital energy. As the opening simile of the text announces, Spain's chastity,
its virginity, is the immutable sign of its eternal purity and health
despite the contemporarily debilitating, but ultimately salubrious
state of illness described in the *Idearium español*. In this light Nietzsche's amendment of Ariston's stoic motto could be re-written as
follows for the *Idearium español*, "*Spain*'s virtue is the health of *her*
soul." For although Ganivet extensively records what he perceives
as the symptoms of political, national weakness and intellectual illness at both the individual and collective level, such symptoms are
only the superficial manifestations of momentary conflict with the
deeper, underlying and eternal territorial spirit. Spain's debilitation
is due to the transgression of virtue, the loss of vital internal energies and the violation of the Virgin, the metaphors for European ex-
pansionism, New World colonialism and capitalist modernization.
Yet this debilitation has not changed the territorial spirit as Spain
finds itself "a la vejez con el espíritu virgen." Spain's illness, then, is
a sign of a greater underlying health, a kind of immunological reaction to *foreign* ideas. Ganivet's clinical discussion of aboulia voices
just such an idea. Significantly, the symptoms of aboulia are accen-
tuated when the sufferer is confronted with new ideas. Specifically,

the primary abulic dysfunctions of association, and more importantly of assimilation, become more acute in the face of modern, non-Spanish ideas: "Los síntomas intelectuales de la abulia son muchos: la atención se debilita tanto más cuanto más *nuevo o extraño* es el objeto sobre el cual hay que fijarla; el entendimiento parece como que se petrifica y se incapacita para la *asimilación* de *ideas nuevas*:..." (my italics 163). The new idea is displaced by the *idée fixe* and ends in the previously discussed "impulsión violenta."

Aboulia, then, is the final stage in a curative illness which disabuses Spain of its imitative fascination with ideas foreign to its natural territorial interests, an assertion which reverses the polarity of the conventional understanding of national inferiority or superiority:

> Ni las ideas francesas, ni las inglesas, ni las alemanas, ni las que puedan más tarde estár en boga, nos sirven, porque nosotros, aunque inferiores en cuanto a la influencia política, somos superiores, más adelantados en cuanto al punto en que se halla nuestra natural evolución; por el hecho de perder sus fuerzas dominadoras (y todas las naciones han de llegar a perderlas), nuestra nación ha entrado en una nueva fase de su vida histórica y ha de ver cuál dirección le está marcada por sus intereses actuales y por sus tradiciones. (157-8)

Here Ganivet inscribes the abulic rejection of foreign and fashionable ideas within the greater dynamic of the evolution of the territorial ideal. Although materially weak, Spain is more evolved than other nations in that it has returned to its essential purity while other nations must still work through their layers of superficial, historical distraction.

For Ganivet, Spain's essential purity is in part proven by the very material impotence that others describe as the source or symptom of its illness. Importantly, Ganivet does not point to Spain's relative economic backwardness as an index of its sickness. On the contrary, Spain's poverty, like its illness, becomes a virtue in the *Idearium español*. Ganivet's valorization of poverty borrows from the Christian ascetic tradition in its rejection of material and corporal pleasure. According to this logic economic development, particularly through the private accumulation of wealth, is viewed as an immoral, sensual enterprise. Ganivet fictionalizes his co-functional valorization of chastity and poverty in *Los trabajos del infatigable creador Pío Cid* when Cortés, anticipating the same argument elaborated in the *Idearium español*, explains to Pío Cid that Spain's inability to profit from the conquest is a sign of spiritual superiority: "Los grandes pueblos y los grandes hombres, pobres han sido y serán; y las empresas más grandiosas son aquellas en que no interviene el dinero, en que los gastos recaen exclusivamente sobre el cerebro y el corazón" (Ginsberg 61). Here the spiritual superiority of poverty is clearly associated with the repression of the corporal, all that which is not "cerebro y corazón," in that both are divorced from the corrupting influences of money and the lower half of the body.

This negative association between the money and the body is expressed in the *Idearium español* regarding projects of modernization and development. Ganivet felt that such projects threatened the traditional culture, social relations and craftsmanship of his idealized image of a pre-industrial Spain. As Lily Litvak has demonstrated at great length, Ganivet was not alone in his opposition to the effects of what she has termed "industrial civilization" in Spain. In the works of Ganivet, Unamuno, Azorín, Valle-Inclán and others the underlying connections between the reappraisal of handicrafts, the daily life or intrahistory of the masses, tradition and narrative instances of *costumbrismo* were posited in opposition to industrial civilization. In all of his works Ganivet vehemently criticized the dehumanizing and fragmenting effects of technological innovations (he opposed the introduction of electricity and running water into his hometown of Granada) and mass production. Ganivet feared for the skilled and independent artisan who worked, according to Ganivet's social fantasy, out of vocation as much as necessity. Ganivet criticizes this transformation of the artisan from independent skilled laborer to unskilled and exploited worker in the *Idearium español* when he discusses the shift from shoe-maker to shoe factory:

> Venimos pues, a la misma conclusión que cuando hablábamos del propietario: hay un obrero socialment útil, el que trabaja y ama su obra, y un obrero perjudicial, el que trabaja por instinto utilitario. Esto no lo dice sólo la cabeza: meditando un poco sobre el caso del zapatero, paréceme que hasta nuestros pies se pondrían de parte de la ya extinguida descendencia de San

Crispín, quien nunca trabajó en ninguna fábrica, ni hubiera lle-
gado a ser santo si hubiera sido fabricante. (83)

In this passage Ganivet associates the lack of industrialization
and large-scale commerce with saintliness and purity; Spain's industrial and commercial impotence becomes a national virtue. Here
the virtue of pre-industrial labor, championed by the figure of San
Crispín, is determined through its association with a non-profit mo-
tivation or use value whereas the original sin of the socially debilitating "obrero perjudicial" is his purely monetary or utilitarian mo-
tivation. Ganivet's moral rejection of exchange value is based upon
his denunciation of property in general. In the *Idearium español* he
rejects both individual and collective property, only recognizing the
spiritual "love," or use value of an individual home-owner for the
ancestral home "porque en ella nació y piensa morir," as opposed
to the landlord who builds, buys and sells dangerously shoddy
homes for profit. Ganivet goes on to summarize his critique of
property by condemning "modern progress" in general as the replacement of use value or "propiedad fija," defined as that which
serves to "atender a las necesidades del vivir," with exchange value
or "propiedad móvil," the continual exchange of capital designed
to meet the needs of financial "strategy" and not social "justice."

Confronted with the brutal commercial leveling of capitalism
and industrialization, and lacking the "ideas céntricas" to propose
nationally concordant alternatives, Ganivet posits a plan of negative
or absent action. The specific terms which Ganivet uses to describe
his project of non-involvement are "withdrawal," and more importantly, "abstention." In choosing this non-participatory path to
power Ganivet seeks to lay claim to the authority and dignity invested in the figure of the ascetic priest. Such a move is anticipated by
the text's positioning of the Virgin and Seneca (complete with his
"hoja de parra"), two formidable figures of abstinence, at the symbolic core of the text. The omnipresence of the previously discussed
chaste and stoic discourses throughout the *Idearium español* give a
definitively *sexual* overtone to the notion of national abstinence or
withdrawal. In this sense the retiring ideal of abstinence from sexual
and material life which Ganivet projects on to Spain is non-produc-
tive, reflecting a pre- or non-capitalist social configuration. The disuse of sexuality is equivalent to the disuse of a productive mode in
that a society must maintain a high level of (re)production in order

to stimulate consumption. The notion of abstinence at work in the *Idearium español*, which rejects both mass-production and mass-gratification, belongs to a pre-capitalist ideology of the body.

At the national level a program of abstinence fits in with the paradigm of national illness. Spain, Ganivet asserts, is in a state of "convalecencia" from its previous overseas excesses and is in no condition to undertake new expansionist enterprises. In fact Ganivet implicitly links abstention to aboulia, positing the former as a means of transforming the listless passivity and indecision of the latter into a form of affirmative action; he states: "Quien no tiene fuerzas bastantes para decidir,..." a description of aboulia, "está obligado a trabajar porque no se decida nada; y si la solución está pendiente porque los intereses se hallan en el equilibrio, lo más sabio y al mismo tiempo lo más cómodo es la abstención" (141). In other words, the only dignified course of action in the face of inevitable embarrassing and humiliating failure is "el retraimiento voluntario" (139).

At this point it is necessary to return to Ganivet's assertion that aboulia is a disorder of assimilation. Abstinence is a compensatory manifestation of aboulia or degeneration which transforms the stigma of impotence into the decisiveness of willful withdrawal. Specifically, theories of degeneration center around the racial, cultural and gender inability or unwillingness to comply with the biological, economic and social demands of existence as defined by the dominant sectors of society. The principal symptom of degeneration-aboulia is the incapacity to concentrate or take action. Abstinence converts this impotence into a form of deliberate will and action. In this sense the discourse of sexual neurosis in the *Idearium español*, aboulia, is an inverted attempt to satisfy the concrete necessities of existence. Thus abstinence is differentiated from degeneration in social terms. [15]

---

[15] As the degeneracy theorist and psychologist Wilhelm Stekel argues in *The Homosexual Neurosis*: "It seems to me that true degeneration, as seen in the stigmata of physical decay, and which manifests itself in an insufficient adjustment to the ethical requirements of society, represents rather the terminal point of an exhausted stem, gravitating downwards, while the neurotic represents a progression." (297)

Here Stekel relates artistic genius with neurosis, a common belief in turn-of-the-century psychoanalysis. Stekel conceives of the neurotic as a social aporia who makes the social restrictions imposed by society stand out in their absolute artificiality. In this sense the neurotic-artists, or the *"dégénérés supérieurs,"* as Stekel called them, recuperate and defend the primary material of human consciousness against the conformist forces of society and culture.

In this sense it is possible to consider how the discourse of illness at work in the *Idearium español* originates in the inability or resistance of the pre-modern or pre-capitalist consciousness to fulfill the requirements of capitalist society. Ganivet, as the voice of a "pre-capitalist" or "underdeveloped" society according to Western standards, articulates the resistance of said society to what Stekel calls "the ethical requirements of society." The requirements of late capitalism consist of an operation of appropriation which replaces the use value of material goods, ideas and sentiments with a market-oriented conception of exchange value. For the pre- or non-capitalist consciousness, that is, for someone who reproduces another code of productive relations, values and behaviors, this utilitarian reduction proves to be vulgar, irreverent, degenerate or *sick*. In the *Idearium español* this conflict is manifested as undifferentiated degeneration or illness. It is undifferentiated to the extent that the social realignment of productive forces and relations provoking this social disarticulation, as well as the resulting symptoms of resistance and lassitude, are both ascribed to a greater process of overdetermined pathology. Aboulia is simultaneously the cause and symptom of the national dilemma. This is the underlying contradiction which informs the text.

For this reason Ganivet promotes abstinence as the solution to the individual and collective dilemma of the nation. Abstinence, as an idealized solution for the sexual neurosis of Ganivet, and as a plan of "ascetic action" for the nation, recuperates the central theme of the text and the *idée fixe* of its author. Specifically, the solution of abstinence reiterates the *Idearium español*'s obsession with the conservation of sexual energy and potency. Beginning with the initial symbol of the Virgin and continuing with "la hoja de parra del senequismo," Ganivet proceeds to tie the past, present and future of Spain to his personal obsessions about sexuality and health. The asceticism of the *Idearium español* relates social and cultural degeneration with the satisfaction of political, material and sexual appetites. In opposition to the physical debilitation which follows from the realization of these appetites (aboulia), Ganivet evokes introspection, virginity, abstinence and sexual repression.

Ganivet's asceticism is nourished by the sexual repression/obsession of the age and his corresponding mission of objective diagnosis. Asceticism, as Nietzsche affirms, is an instrument of power. The negation of the carnal-material world is a tactic for consolidating control over it. The ascetic's inadaptation to the sexual and material demands of society becomes the negation-repression of the same. Through this sexual-material denial, the ascetic negatively complies with these concrete necessities without participating in their realization. In this way the ascetic is not implicated in the vulgarity and inequality of the material and sensual world. The ascetic priest or philosopher seeks to acquire an authority of critical distance which enables him/her to have a role in the direction and control of the reproduction of the material world. In this sense Ganivet offers himself as a spiritual priest or doctor for Spain, while he also projects Spain as a materially disinterested "parent" for Latin America.

In the *Idearium español* Ganivet posits an asceticism based on a kind of sexual-material nihilism. His revulsion of the material, corporal and sensual elements of life expresses his will to nothingness. Incapable of complying with the requisites of capitalist interpellation, Ganivet prefers to repose in abstraction and nothingness, the philosophical outcome of the death of God, a path not uncommon at the turn of the century as indicated by Nietzsche in *On the Genealogy of Morals*:

> We can no longer conceal from ourselves *what* is expressed by all that willing which has taken its direction from the ascetic ideal: this hatred of the human, and even more of the animal, and more still of the material, this horror of the senses, of reason itself, this fear of happiness and beauty, this longing to get away from all appearance, change, becoming, death wishing, from longing itself – all this means – let us dare to grasp it – *a will to nothingness*, an aversion to life, a rebellion against the most fundamental presuppositions of life; but it remains a *will*! (162)

Once again the importance of faith and disillusionment stands out in the functioning of the text. As with geographical-racial determinism and the metaphysics of the national soul, the will to nothingness is premised upon the loss of faith. The functioning of the text, in particular its determinist argument, rests on the negated manifestation of God, nothingness. In this notion the incapacity of sexual-material gratification converges with the flight to chaste and ahistorical abstraction. Through pure abstraction the text seeks to establish a space free from material-carnal contamination, or in other words, free from history. Ganivet returns to the period of pre-history in order to recover personal and national innocence. In the *Idearium español* he creates a pre-history of sacred symbols whose mythological essence resists the corruption of the biological and historical impulse.

Thus Ganivet, anticipating Freud and Marcuse, also linked the tension between biological urgency and psychological repression on the one hand, with the antagonism between the historical and mythological interpretation of a civilization on the other. Ganivet and Spain regress to the mythological womb of pre-history in the acorporal symbol of the Virgin. Through this symbol Ganivet seeks the gratification of nothingness, of pre-existence. In this way the Spanish soul embodied in Ganivet, achieves the pleasure of non-existence, a state as divine as it is nihilist.

The *Idearium español* documents the search for and formulation of the consciousness of an individual, Ganivet, within the greater discursive project of national analysis and consciousness-raising. This attempt at self and national constitution characterizes the ideological tension which motivates the intellectual positions of the text. The negation of the connections between the concrete and the abstract in human experience is established as an interpretive frame and narrative of the Spanish soul. Insofar as this break or discontinuity is experienced and perceived as an illness, the philosophical split between the ideal and the material becomes embedded in a narrative of diagnosis and cure. This clinical narrative reappears in the oppositions between the material and the spiritual, the libidinal and the ideal, and the historical and the mythological. Specifically, the autobiographical and national vision of the text derives from intellectual-psychological inhibition; from the inability or aversion to associate the material with the abstract, the libidinal with the ideal. In the *Idearium español* an ideological aversion becomes a model for analysis. Through this analysis the text corrects the past, devalues the present and prescribes the future.

The stagnation and inhibition of the collective subject of the *Idearium español* finds its intellectual complement in geographical-racial determinism, while it finds its philosophical complement in the introspective metaphysics of the national soul. In this way the inability to associate the material and the abstract has both scientific and metaphysical foundations. The union of these psychically conditioned and intellectually determinist visions leads the text to a

paralyzing dissociation. Ironically, it is this mental paralysis which
Ganivet diagnoses as the national illness:

> Como la falta de apetito material denota una disminuición de la
> actividad digestiva, así también la falta de apetito espiritual,
> manifestada en la desidia de las facultades que actúan exterior-
> mente, revela una debilitación de esa energía asimiladora interna
> que los aristotélicos llamaban entendimiento agente y los posi-
> tivistas sentido sintético, que no es otra cosa que la inteligencia
> misma funcionando según la ley de asociación. Así, pues, la
> causa de la abulia es, a mi juicio, la debilitación del sentido sin-
> tético, de la facultad de asociar las representaciones. (135)

Degeneration, as a concept manifested under the term of *aboulia* in the *Idearium español*, and as an intellectual concept of the age,
simultaneously develops within an internal history of ideas and in
relation to radical material changes of the period. Degeneration, as
a symbolic obsession of the period, documents the disintegration of
a socio-cultural system and the emergence of another. The constitu-
tive ideologies of the period could not keep up with its extensive
and rapid material and social transformations. There emerged a gap
between technological "progress" and the mental capacity of per-
ceiving and assimilating the same. Sensations of malaise or confusion or *aboulia* are not the objective causes or symptoms of a social
"malady," but rather constitute the dominant subjective epistemological frame for narrating the gap between the economic, social
and political reorganization of society and humanity's or a specific
culture's ability to comprehend and reproduce such changes.

Paradoxically, Ganivet's discourse of national infirmity works
within the bourgeois discursive practice of publicly erasing its class
interest. Ganivet proposes, in an introspective and ahistorical
prose, an intra-history of symbols, images and myths which transcend the limitations of class; which transcend the restrictions of his
interpellation as a bourgeois subject. The aboulia and impotence
which are first described as a national illness, also constitute a
virtue of aristocratic-ascetic abstinence from sexuality, economics
and history. The fact that Spain has not industrialized is simultaneously its proof of virginity, acorporeality, ahistoricity and the confused statement of an intellectual simultaneously defining the material impotence of his nation as sickness and purity.

This chaste and ahistorical vision of the *Idearium español* underscores a conceptual matrix which combines apparently conflicting
ideas about sexuality and capitalism. The concept of aboulia, a dysfunctional abstinence from the material and the corporal provoked
by impotence, narrates Ganivet's ideological resistance to capitalist
subject interpellation. Ganivet rejects the logic of capitalist culture.
His sexual neurosis is also a social and political protest. Ganivet
maintains his psychological formation against the new cultural con-
formity and coercion of mass production and consumption. In
these psychological terms, Ganivet is, to borrow a phrase from Wilhelm Stekel: "a revolutionary who does not inwardly recognize the
laws of culture" (*Compulsion* 38). The code of socio-cultural values
preserved by Ganivet clash with those of the new capitalist code.
Capitalism strips away the aura of the object/concept in order to
reinvent it as a commodity or property. As Ganivet states:

> La propiedad intelectual está fundada sobre un error profundo.
> Cuando el trabajo del hombre se inspira en la idea de lucro, bien
> es que le estimule mediante el interés personal; pero es incon-
> gruente aplicar el mismo principio a las obras de la ciencia o del
> arte, las cuales no deben de tener otro motivo de inspiración que
> el amor a la verdad o a la belleza. Conceder patentes de inven-
> ción a un sabio o a un artista es convertirles en industriales de la
> ciencia o del arte, exitarles a que conviertan sus obras en artícu-
> los de comercio. (99)

With the commercialization of goods, services and ideas under
capitalism, and more importantly, with the subsequent professionalization of intellectuals and academic institutions, their accompanying philosophies are re-organized around the demands of capital. In
this scenario the merit of aesthetic ideas or products and socio-cultural practices is reduced to their exchange value.

The closing thoughts of the *Idearium español* reiterate Ganivet's
resistance to the increasing commodification of life in a way which
seeks to recuperate Spain's inability to compete politically and economically, namely its illness, as a self-imposed program of purifica-
tion and penance which will enable it to return to international
prominence:

> Hemos de hacer un acto de contrición colectiva; hemos de des-
> doblarnos, aunque muchos nos quedamos en tan arriesgada

operación, y así tendremos pan espiritual para nosotros y nuestra familia, que lo anda mendigando por el mundo, y nuestras conquistas materiales podrán ser aún fecundas, porque al renacer hallaremos una inmensidad de pueblos hermanos a quienes marcar con el sello de nuestro espíritu. (148)

This act of collective penance summarizes the contradictory metaphysical and moral obsessions which constitute the argument of the *Idearium español*. Ganivet ends the text with an evocation which interprets the material and spiritual suffering of Spain as a self-imposed punishment. The very notion that there is something to atone for once again invokes the recurrent theme of original sin introduced in the opening simile of the Virgin and the violation of the national spirit. Spain must humble itself to atone for its sexual-national transgressions against the true territorial spirit, posited in the guise of a violated yet pure image of woman. Such contrition will ennoble an otherwise sickly state of national prostration and facilitate an economic and political recovery at home and abroad. Here Ganivet at once associates and disassociates the ideal from the material and the spiritual from the corporal in a contradictory movement which is characteristic of the text. Spain must mortify its material, political and sexual body in order to regain spiritual health. Yet it is this negation of the sexual-material which will permit Spain to return to economic, political and colonial enterprises in the future. Importantly, he refers to such enterprises as "nuestras conquistas materiales," a phrasing which legitimizes colonial practices which he had previously denounced in the text. Moreover, he refers to these "conquistas" as "fecundas," once again lending them a tone of sexual possession or violence which results in "pueblos hermanos" who are marked "con el sello de nuestro espíritu." In this way the *Idearium español* ends with the same mixture of spiritual purity and sexual violence with which it begins. This mixture functions within the confused series of complementary oppositions which inform the text, simultaneously proclaiming Spain to be superior and inferior, spiritual and sensual, healthy and sick.

CHAPTER 2

JOSÉ ENRIQUE RODÓ'S *ARIEL:* THE THERAPEUTIC PROGRAM FOR PAN-AMERICAN RECOVERY

ARIEL AND THE ORGANICIST MODEL OF NATIONAL HEALTH

José Enrique Rodó's *Ariel* (1900) was written at a time of profound international, national and personal crisis. The Hispanic world had only recently witnessed and directly experienced the defeat and replacement of a generally remote, incompetent and decrepit colonial power, Spain, at the hands of a seemingly vibrant and dangerously close political threat, the United States. The 1898 transferal of Spain's remaining colonial possessions, Cuba, Puerto Rico and the Philippines, to North American control abruptly transformed any Latin American admiration for its northern neighbor into suspicion and anxiety concerning national sovereignty and self-determination.

At the national level *Ariel* appeared in Uruguay during the period of the military regimes of Latorre and Santos (Concha 124), civil war and modernization characterized by radically opposing polemics and proposals, a political and rhetorical intolerance Rodó denounced as "jacobinismo." Rodó's prognosis for the nation's ills was pessimistic if not nihilistic: "Nada hay de seguro en nuestro país, ni en política, ni en cuestión económica; todo es inestable, problemático, todo está amenazado de mil peligros y expuesto a desaparecer de la noche a la mañana: incluso el país mismo" (Lazo XX).

At the personal level Rodó seems to have experienced one of his periodic bouts with depression, pessimism and anxiety around the time of the publication of *Ariel* (Concha 124). As a committed national and pan-American educator, author and politician Rodó's personal crises cannot be clearly separated from the larger social problems afflicting turn-of-the-century Uruguay. Like Ganivet, in his personal correspondence he drew an analogy between his own psychic exhaustion and the ongoing political conflict in his country. In a letter to his friend Francisco Piquet Rodó states that the turmoil caused by civil strife had left him and the nation "exhaustos, esquilmados y pelados" (Lazo XX).

Out of this personal and collective sense of fatigue and decadence comes *Ariel*, a strikingly optimistic program for pan-American regeneration. The appeal to a broader, extra-national cultural constituency reflected Rodó's moral and intellectual disenchantment with the Uruguayan political parliamentary (or "charlamentario" as he called it) system. In this sense the double discourse of degeneration/regeneration employed in *Ariel* represents a cultural pan-American "nationalism" rather than a championing of a specific Uruguayan nationalism or national identity. As John Beverley maintains of *modernismo*'s pan-American approach to the intertwined issues of modernization, cultural autonomy and imperialism in general:

> The movement was cosmopolitan, francophile, bohemian, pan-American (in the sense that the *modernistas* sought to write for a general rather than national reading public); it stressed the separation of art from politics and commerce, the power of fantasy and the imagination, sensuality, the idealization of the past, above all the careful cultivation and enrichment of poetic language and form itself. (*Literature* 54)

In this context, unlike Ganivet's *Idearium español* and Arguedas' *Pueblo enfermo*, Rodó's *Ariel* does not specifically examine the ills of Uruguay in particular, but rather addresses the need for a "universal," Latin American renewal.

As in Ganivet, this perceived need of regeneration, implicitly has as its precondition the perception of a state of degeneration or decadence. For although Rodó does not explicitly qualify Latin America as "degenerate" or "sick" like other Latin American thinkers of his day, the symbolism inherent in the Ariel-Caliban opposition itself indicates that he is less confident about the contemporary state of Latin American "health" than he is about its hypothesized, therapeutic future.

The threats to Latin American health discussed in *Ariel* are both internal and external to the Latin American "body-politic." In a synthesis that has proved to be extremely provocative for the text's reception, both the internal and external sources of disease are personified in the symbol and body of Caliban. Caliban simultaneously fulfills many symbolic roles. Firstly, he represents the foreign political and cultural threat posed by the United States, as evidenced by its increased intervention in Latin America. Secondly, Caliban gives specific physiological and symbolic form to turn-of-the-century elite fears regarding sexual, racial and social leveling and mixing, fears fueled in turn by theories of evolution, sexology, pathology and psychology which maintained democracy's alleged tendency to inhibit natural selection and thus weaken the species. In fact, this apparently contradictory double significance of Caliban in Rodó's appropriation of the symbol is reciprocally reinforcing.[16] For although Caliban undeniably refers to a foreign political threat, the greatest danger posed by the United States in *Ariel* is the attractiveness of its economic and political model for the youth of Latin America. It is this anxiety surrounding the vulnerability of Latin America's youth – a potential source of internal debility and enervation – which preoccupies Rodó in *Ariel*.

Rodó addresses his concern about emulating the North American model through his reading of the psycho-pathological theories of personality proposed by Walter Bagehot in *Physics and Politics* of 1872 and Jean Gabrielle Tarde in *Les lois de l'imitation* of 1890 (Brotherston 72). Rodó's theories of psychological imitation centering around the normal or abnormal formation of an integral, healthy individual personality are extrapolated onto society, thus constituting a metaphorical model of mental function or disfunction for society. This attraction to the North American model is in itself diagnosed as a psychological disorder of imitation, "nordo-

---

[16] It is important to note that Rodó was not the first Latin American intellectual to deflect the degenerative onus of Caliban away from Latin America and onto the United States. In 1898 the Franco-Argentinean writer Paul Groussac declared: "desde la Secesión y la brutal invasión del Oeste, se ha desprendido libremente el espíritu yankee del cuerpo informe y 'calibanesco', y el viejo mundo ha contemplado con inquietud y terror a la novísima civilización que pretende suplantar a la nuestra declarada caduca." Quoted in José Enrique Rodó, *Obras completas*, edition, introduction, notes and prologue by Emir Rodríguez Monegal (Madrid, 1957), p. 193.

manía," a condition analogous to a mental disease or disorder, as indicted by the suffix -manía.

In this sense the degenerative threat posed by the figure of Caliban is both external and internal to Latin American political, cultural and social health. This interplay between internal and external irritants or infectious agents in the national "body" is basic to the disease paradigm of nineteenth century socio-political thought borrowed from the medical and natural sciences. Rodó is approximating the external versus internal etiology of biological and *social* disease proposed by Rudolf Virchow in *Cellular Pathology* (1858). As Sander Gilman has affirmed, Virchow compared the structure of the state to different biological organisms:

> For Virchow the interaction of the cells in the body was equivalent to the interaction of citizens in the body politic. Disease arose from only two sources: an active external source ("irritation") and a passive internal source. The latter he labeled "degeneration." So within the human body as well as within the body politic forces are constantly at work which expose hidden weaknesses of the body and can cause eventual collapse. ("Sexology" 73)

Ariel, despite its overtly spiritualist and aestheticist rhetoric, is firmly rooted in the social organicist analogy between biological and social systems. In fact, Rodó's spiritual and scientific discourses are complementary constituents of an encompassing aesthetization of biological and evolutionary theory. In a poetic mixture of biology, theology, psychology and the social sciences, Rodó approximates Virchow's micro-biological and cellular analogy for social systems. The following passage from *Ariel* suggests, for example, a "cellular" basis for the coexistence of the unrecognized yet dignified masses and the maintenance of a cultural elite, an *"aristarquia,"* [sic] within democracy:

> ...las afirmaciones de la ciencia contribuyen a sancionar y fortalecer en la sociedad el espíritu de la democracia, revelando cuánto es el valor natural del esfuerzo colectivo; cuál la grandeza de la obra de los pequeños: cuán inmensa la parte de acción reservada al colaborador anónimo y oscuro en cualquiera manifestación del desenvolvimiento universal. Realiza, no menos que la revelación cristiana, la dignidad de los humildes, esta nueva revelación

atribuye, en la naturaleza, a la obra de los infinitamente pequeños, a la labor del nummulite y el briozoo en el fondo oscuro
del abismo, la construcción de los cimientos geológicos; que
hace surgir la vibración de la célula informe y primitiva, todo el
impulso ascendente de las formas orgánicas; que manifiesta el
poderoso papel que en nuestra vida psíquica es necesario
atribuir a los fenómenos más inaparentes y vagos... y que llegan-
do a la sociología y a la historia, restituye el heroísmo, a menudo
abnegado, de las muchedumbres,... (33)

Here the Christian embrace of the meek becomes the undetected
existence of microscopic organisms, the bryozoans who labor in the
depths of a prehistoric sea towards the formation of "higher" evolutionary, social and cultural forms, "el impulso ascendente de las
formas orgánicas," otherwise known as the "aristarquia."

Rodó's constant application of the jargon of evolution and natural selection to social and cultural history is perhaps the strongest
and most irrefutable evidence of his reliance on the biological social
organicist model. Rodó openly attributes his employment of the
natural sciences in his evaluation of social and cultural development
to the influence of such seminal degeneracy theorists as Auguste
Comte, Herbert Spencer, Hippolyte Taine and Jean-Marie Guyau.

In a curious passage in *Ariel* Rodó even makes passing reference
to Comte's reliance on the science of phrenology, a discipline for
distinguishing the normal or healthy brain and skull from the abnormal or diseased specimen:

> El empequeñecimiento de un cerebro humano por el comercio
> continuo de un solo modo de actividad, es para Comte un re-
> sultado comparable a la mísera suerte del obrero a quien la
> división de trabajo de taller le obliga a consumir en la inva-
> riable operación de un detalle mecánico todas las energías de
> su vida. (11)

The passage suggests another evolutionary model which competed
with Darwin's theory of natural selection. Rodó attributes the reduction in brain size to the dull routine and subsequent physiological atrophy of mass production, which is an evolutionary change
provoked from outside of the internal history of the species. This is
an example of the Lamarckian concept of evolutionary adaptation
to environmental conditions and not the natural selection of the most

suited species to a given environment. [17] Since the Lamarckian view of evolution (as opposed to Darwin's) allows for the genetic transmission of such acquired traits, it is an ominous notion for degeneracy theorists in that it allows for circumstantially generated pathologies, (in Rodó's passage the mentally and anatomically debilitating effects of mechanized labor), to be passed on to future generations. [18]

Rodó's connection to a Lamarckian theory of socio-biological adaptation and evolution is further evidenced by his references to the work of Herbert Spencer. Spencer's works in social psychology and biology were foundational to the development of Social Darwinism in the nineteenth century. In such works as *Social Statistics* (1850), *Principles of Psychology* (1855) and *First Principles* (1862), Spencer viewed society as an organism undergoing a process of evolution similar and related to the biological model. Spencer made use of the phrenology of Carl Vogt and Franz Joseph Gall, linking brain measurement and other physiological signs to the evolution and differentiation of the human species (Dijkstra 166). Of further importance to a consideration of Rodó's psychologically and biologically oriented construction of pan-American identity, Spencer tied his methodological dependence on empirical individualism to collective ethnic or national experience by conceptualizing a unified racial evolutionary experience (Nye 56). According to this theory, the inherent physical and mental properties of a "race" interact with specific environmental conditions, producing generationally transmissible anatomical and psychic traits which could have either a progressive or regressive evolutionary outcome. In this sense Spencer is clearly allied with the degeneracy theorists of the period who were anxious about social contradictions of the natural order.

Another significant manifestation of Rodó's alignment with the organicist school is his description of the work of Hippolyte Taine.

---

[17] For a comparison of Darwin's and Lamarck's theories of evolution see Robert A. Nye, "Sociology: The Irony of Progress," *Degeneration: The Dark Side of Progress*, Eds. J. Edward Chamberlin and Sander L. Gilman (New York: Columbia Univ. Press, 1985), 57.

[18] In his *The Division of Labor in Society* (1893), the French sociologist Emile Durkheim proposed the Lamarckian-based theory that the division of labor effects the brain and the nervous system in an adaptive response to the increased pace and complexity of production. For a discussion of Durkheim's neuropathological theory, see Nye, 60.

This reference to Taine is typical of Rodó's expository method in
Ariel wherein he repeatedly cites the work of renowned authors as
a kind of corroborative shorthand for his own less rigorously or explicitly advanced theories; Rodó writes:

> En cuanto a Taine, es quien ha escrito los *Orígenes de la Francia
> contemporánea* y si, por una parte, su concepción de la sociedad
> como un organismo, le conduce lógicamente a rechazar toda
> idea de uniformidad que se oponga al principio de las dependen-
> cias y las subordinaciones orgánicas, por otra parte su finísimo
> instinto de selección natural le lleva a abominar de la invasión de
> las cumbres por la multitud. (29)

Not only does Rodó's admiring synopsis of Taine's ideas point to its
organicist origin, but he also goes on to link their shared analogy of
the state as organism to its logical corollary that social ideas and
movements that oppose the "natural" biological order of society,
such as social, racial and sexual egalitarianism, threaten to impose
an unhealthy state of socio-biological homogenization on a normally self-differentiating natural world.

   Jean-Marie Guyau is another influence on Rodó directly tied to
degeneracy theory. Guyau's literary and social criticism was princi-
pally concerned with investigating the discourse of the 'mal du siècle' associated with decadent literature. As F.J.W. Harding affirms,
Guyau characterized the texts and literary sensibilities of decadence
as pathological, linking the very poetic and narrative structures of
these writings with the disorganized thoughts of the criminal or insane mind (94-95). Such symptoms of literary pathology were not
only deemed by Guyau to be of individual origin but were indicative of the degeneration of an entire nation or race.

   In addition to Rodó, there are other citations which register the
dissemination of Guyau's degeneracy theory among certain segments in Latin American literature and criticism. In the case of
Rubén Darío the reaction to such medical criticism was negative.
Darío described Guyau in medical terms: "Guyau, el admirable y
joven sabio, sacrificó en las aras de los nuevos ídolos científicos. El
comprobó, como un profesor que toma el pulso, el estado patológi-
co de su edad, el progreso de fiebre moral siempre en crecimiento"
(451).

   Whereas Darío rejected Guyau's criticism as a practice of "au-
topsia espiritual," Rodó was attracted to the moralizing anthropo-

morphism of his theory. [19] One of Guyau's theories that would have
resonance in *Ariel* is the belief that the stages of regeneration and
degeneration of a race are akin to the periods of youth and old age
in the individual. In *Ariel*, Rodó discusses the cyclic rejuvenation of
youth in a strange, misogynistic anecdote he attributes to Guyau. In
this story the hope and vitality of youth is compared to an insane
and jilted bride who suffers daily disappointment, yet continues to
await her groom with renewed hope every morning. The moral
beauty of the story, its "conmovedora locura," is the act of self-
willed faith which allows the deceived bride to awaken fresh every
day, put on her gown and veil and say to herself "Es hoy cuando
vendrá." This passage lends an affirmative function to female psy-
chosis in which it serves the greater good of male regeneration.
After all, for Guyau and Rodó, what else would this imaginary, de-
ranged woman have to do with her time other than aid in the renewal of masculine virility, the foundation of national health. In this
case, pathology, so widely feared when present in men, i.e. society,
is quite normal if not functional when manifest in women.

Further substantiating Rodó's organicist interpretation of social
organization, and more importantly, social conflicts, are subsequent
references to an unnamed "pensador ilustre" who described slavery
as "una partícula no digerida por el organismo social" (50); and to
Edgard Quinet who "tan profundamente ha penetrado en las armonías de la historia y la naturaleza..." (54). Given *Ariel*'s dense intertextual relationship with the literary, scientific, philosophical,
psychological and sociological texts of the period, it is sometimes
difficult to isolate specific examples of organicist or degeneracy theory that are not tied to some direct or indirect outside reference.
Yet there are instances in the text wherein Rodó independently employs organicist and clinical rhetoric which provide us with an
index of the degree to which he internalized these theories. As was
previously stated, Rodó's use of evolutionary discourse throughout

---

[19] Darío's complaint that Guyau performed "spiritual autopsy" on authors
could also be applied to Darío himself. On the occasion of Oscar Wilde's death
Darío critically dissected Wilde, a victim of the discourse of degeneration and ho-
mophobia, comparing his dead body to that of a dead and infectious dog. In this in-
stance Darío embraces the criticism of literary pathology which he dislikes in
Guyau. For a discussion of Darío's literary obituary of Wilde see Sylvia Molloy,
"Too Wilde for Comfort: Desire and Ideology in Fin-de-Siècle Spanish America,"
Social Text 31/32 (1992): 189-190.

Ariel is the most basic and undeniable evidence of his bio-clinical foundation, yet for those who would attribute this to mere discursive fashion there are other more direct expressions of the biological paradigm. At times, Rodó explicitly, and without reference to an outside authority, compares social institutions to an organism. Rodó calls the United States "un inmenso organismo nacional" and "aquel titánico organismo social" and describes the modern city as "un organismo necesario de la alta cultura."

The belief that society and social institutions are analogous to an organism inexorably involves the analysis of society and its institutions in terms of the "health" of the organism. Within this analogy many different medical metaphors are possible including those of circulation, respiration, vitality, and anatomical integrity, differentiation and function. Yet all of these lead to diagnoses of social health along a normal/abnormal or healthy/sick axis. In *Ariel* these scientific metaphors are written into a lofty, stylishly rhetorical, aesthetic discourse which softens the harsh contours of the divide between the normal and the pathological. If we consider Rodó's application of the science of craniology in *Ariel*, we observe just such a softening of a violently differentiating discipline. Craniology and evolutionary theory borrowed from one another, linking the progress of the species to racial and sexual differentiation. Such distinctions were far from our current theoretical notions of "difference" and were based on allegedly measurable variances in quantity and quality. Spencer, anticipating Rodó, made clear the racial and gender-based distinctions of inferiority and superiority based on skull-size and other anatomical measurements:

> evolution is marked by an increasing heterogeneity in the vertebral column, and especially in the components of the skull: the higher forms being distinguished by the relatively larger size of the bones which cover the brain, and the relatively smaller size of those which form the jaws, etc. Now this trait which is stronger in Man than in any other creature, is stronger in the European than in the savage. (Dijkstra 166)

Criminologists such as Cesare Lombroso would build upon the ethnographic and gender basis of craniology and the anatomical stigmata of difference to lend it the added element of criminal deviancy as well. Thus women, criminals, and the non-white races were deemed to be regressive, degenerate or sickly. It is in this historical context that we should consider the following passage from *Ariel*:

> El pensamiento se conquistará, palmo a palmo, por su propia espontaneidad, todo el espacio de que se necesite para afirmar y consolidar su reino, entre las demás manifestaciones de la vida. El, en la organización individual, levanta y engrandece, con su actividad continuada, la bóveda del cráneo que le contiene. Las razas pensadoras revelan, en la capacidad creciente de sus cráneos, ese empuje del obrero interior. (54)

What is at first described as an unaligned abstract principal of thought actualizing itself through its own dynamic is quickly relegated its assigned role as agent for the advancement of the "thinking," or in social darwinist terms, white male "races." In this instance intellectual potential, physiological structure and evolution are intertwined in the over-determined trajectory of the symbol of Ariel, "el imperio de la razón," the pinnacle of the masculine ideal, the chaste winged figure of triumph over the earth-mother and body, and the final manifestation of evolutionary racial superiority. Excluded from this evolutionary fantasy is the figure of Caliban, the "símbolo de sensualidad y torpeza," the incarnation of social effeminization, socio-sexual anarchy and racial inferiority doomed to evolutionary reversion or degeneration.

This phrenological model of psychological evolution and species differentiation, here symbolized by the Ariel/Caliban opposition, inevitably activates the social, sexual and racial tensions and antagonisms implicit in the phrenological model and historically present in turn-of-the-century Latin America. Caliban, the indigenous Latin American, represents the sensual, the effeminate (forever associated with his earth-mother Sycorax) and the degenerate threat to Latin American health, whereas Ariel represents the aryan male regeneration of the Americas.

Believing that the social health and future of Latin America were at stake, Rodó endeavored to produce a program for national revival based on the contrasting psycho-physiological health and pathology of the human body. The Shakespearean figure and symbolic namesake of the Rodó's text, Ariel, the "genio del aire," itself corresponds to an eighteenth-century scientific model for health and illness based on the circulation and revitalizing properties of fresh air and aeration. Alain Corbin has stated apropos of this school of aerist theory: "Definitions of the healthy and unhealthy were sketched out and norms established in terms of aerist thought. The need for ventilation was already being formulated, and the poetic hymn to the purging power of the storm was taking shape" (14). If this were not a description of an eighteenth-century theory of pneumatic chemistry one could mistake it for a summary of the meteorological events of *The Tempest*. What is more significant for a reading of *Ariel* is that Rodó cites the champion of aerist thought, Antoine Lavoisier, as an intellectual martyr of jacobinian terror. This coincidence reinforces the symbolic and physical split between Ariel and Caliban as the dry, purifying and healing air-spirit in opposition to the son of a humid, degenerating earth-mother, referred to in *Ariel* as a "tierra agotada" (Anderson 89-90).

Thus *Ariel* participates in the larger turn-of-the-century iconography of exhaustion. This iconography was binary in character, as manifested by the Ariel-Caliban dichotomy, and centered around notions of virility, emasculation and effeminacy. Within the paradigm of national health, degeneration was linked to the "effeminization" of the national soul and body, a notion which the renowned sexologist Krafft-Ebing made clear in his *Psychopathia Sexualis*: "The episodes of moral decay always coincide with the progression of effeminacy, lewdness and luxurience of the nations" (6).

Such emasculation involved an alleged loss of control over the instinctual, scatological and sexual aspects of human nature, metaphorically expressed through the body as the "lower" instincts or passions. The anxiety regarding the effeminization of society was premised on misogynistic views of women which associated the female with a congenital lack of control over the passions and a biological inability to differentiate sensual from mental experience. The late nineteenth century witnessed a plethora of social scientists, psychologists, sexologists and philosophers who sought to prove this hypothesis through a mixture of supposedly "scientific" empirical studies, evolutionary theory and purely subjective opinion. [20] One of the most influential of these thinkers was Otto Weininger,

---

[20] It would be impossible to give a detailed listing of such texts in the limited space provided here but I will offer a few arbitrary examples to suggest an idea of the output of socio-scientific misogynist literature of the period: Charles Darwin,

who in his study of the sexual-social evolution of the species, *Sex and Character* (1903), postulated that women and the non-white races are limited to corporal or sensual experience and knowledge, a gendered and racial state of being Weininger called the "henid." Weininger qualifies the white male as the only segment of the species capable of differentiating nature, or bodily sensation, from culture, or mental creativity. Inevitably these theories were spatially mapped on the individual and social body in terms of the "lower" instincts, organs, gender and races as opposed to the "higher" Aryan male brain.

Race is an intricate and indistinguishable component in the turn-of-the-century preoccupation with emasculation and degeneration. Race, racial "contamination" and mixing are indistinguishable from the fears surrounding gender and effeminization as suspected causes of degeneration in that from the very beginnings of the evolutionary and phrenological theories of Charles Darwin and Carl Vogt the alleged physiological and mental deficiencies of women and those of the "inferior races" were viewed as nearly identical. In the spiritual or mental realm the non-aryan races were said to share both women's sensual excesses and their inability to control their passions; as George L. Mosse has stated:

> Here it is necessary to point out that the stereotyped depiction of sexual "degenerates" was transformed almost intact to the "inferior races," who inspired the same fears. These races, too, were said to display a lack of morality and a general lack of self discipline. Blacks, and then Jews, were endowed with excessive sexuality, with a so-called female sensuousness that transformed love into lust. They lacked all manliness. (36)

The mastery of these lower, "animal" passions, implicitly associated with the subjugation of the inferior gender and races, was directly connected with notions concerning social, cultural and political discipline, thus linking the self-control of "high-minded" reason to national organization and stability. The health of national institu-

---

The Descent of Man; Paul Mobius, *On the Physiological Debility of Women* (1898); Carl Vogt, *Lectures on Man* (1864); Herbert Spencer, *The Study of Psychology* (1873); Arthur Schopenhauer, "On Women" (1851); Otto Weininger, *Sex and Character* (1903); Cesare Lombroso and Gugliemo Ferrero, *The Female Offender* (1895); Haverlock Ellis, *Man and Woman* (1894).

tions, society and culture was defined in terms of robust, yet continent virility. In this sense the male body and psyche became the model for national discourse concerning the state and national culture. Any threats to, or deficiencies within the nation were perceived of as crises of manhood and resulted in further programs of national regeneration through "re-virilization."

ARIEL AND LATIN AMERICAN HELLENISM

The restorative tonic which Rodó proposed for Latin American youth was a typically nineteenth-century cocktail of virile nationalism, sentimental non-ascetic Christianity and a contradictory combination of sexually charged yet de-eroticized masculine imagery and bonding grounded in the nineteenth-century re-writing of Hellenism. This salubrious and masculine program for continental health answered the challenge of the at once brutally male but vulgarly effeminate utilitarianism of the United States and its political economy of liberal democracy which were incarnated in the ambiguous figure of Caliban. Rodó's Hellenic humanism posited an exclusively masculine agency for national revival, a sentimental grouping which Sylvia Molloy has characterized as a "male bonding *pro patria*" (199). Yet before entering into the specifics of Rodó's Latin American appropriation of the Hellenic model it is necessary to reflect upon the phenomenon of nineteenth-century Hellenism in a wider discursive context.

The resurgence of interest in classical Greece is a complex development of the nineteenth century tied to a rekindled awareness of the body (particularly the male body), a return to nature through images of healing sunlight, invigorating mountain air, rejuvenating physical exercise, and egalitarian nudism. These concepts and practices were conceptually situated in timeless pastoral scenes designed to lend a sense of historical immutability to the very contemporary processes of modernization and the formation of the modern state.

Significantly, these revised classical images were inscribed into the nineteenth century's preoccupation with individual and collective health and regeneration. The emphasis of this *physical* dimension of Hellenism underlined individual and group restoration through renewed contact with nature, strenuous exercise and perhaps most importantly, personal and collective sexual continence. The notion of Hellenic sexual self-control and discipline was a decidedly historical construction of the nineteenth century in alignment with scientifically and philosophically grounded associations between sexual promiscuity and individual and collective enervation. In this sense ancient sensibilities of sexuality were constricted within the nineteenth-century's obsessional censure of the sexual, [21] a repression which was pivotal in the rigidification of gender roles and the classification of homosexuality as a pathological state.

This ideological reformulation of the *physical* dimension of Hellenism points to the disjuncture between the cultural, sexual and social beliefs and practices of antiquity and their reconfiguration in the nineteenth century. Paradoxically, it is the very masculine or virile connotation of classical antiquity, the very quality which is so central to the nineteenth-century discourse of manly nationalism, which provoked great anxiety among the male elite of the period.

In his essay *Rubén Darío*, Rodó distinguished between acceptable and unacceptable Hellenisms. Rodó's version of Hellenism was a de-eroticized construction which emphasized the youth and vitality of ancient Greece. This vision of Hellenism and the importance Rodó attributed to it as a model for social rejuvenation approximated the conservative and homophobic Hellenic ideology of Matthew Arnold in his struggle against Walter Pater and John Addington Symonds in the political infighting at Oxford in the late nineteenth century. [22] Paradoxically, Rodó's notion of the healthy, regenerative role of the Hellenic tradition was voiced by Symonds, the defender of sexual integration and non-heterosexual union in *Studies of the Greek Poets*. In this work Symonds depicts Greece as the embodiment of adolescent health: "A man in perfect health of mind and body, enjoying the balance of mental, moral, and physical qualities

---

[21] When speaking about sexual 'censure' or 'repression' I am referring to the *de facto* prohibition of specific behaviors which was accompanied by a heightened interest and vigilance concerning sexuality. For as Michel Foucault has affirmed in *The History of Sexuality Volume I*, state or familial prohibition of specific practices on medical grounds did not preclude a proliferation of discourses around sexuality but rather accelerated their dissemination.

[22] For a discussion of these sexually and politically charged polemics over the interpretation and dissemination of the Classical tradition at Oxford see Richard Dellamora, "Arnold, Winckelmann and Pater" and "'The New Chivalry' and Oxford Politics" in *Masculine Desire. The Sexual Politics of Victorian Aestheticism* (Chapel Hill: The University of North Carolina Press, 1990).

which health implies, carried within himself the norm and measure of propriety" (Dellamora 162). Rodó's expressed his anxiety concerning this slippage between healthy and sickly views of Hellenism in *Rubén Darío* when he suggests that the modern interpretation of classical myths has been a productive strategy of degenerate or decadent literature: "Los mitos clásicos ¿no son hoy mismo objeto de una tenaz evocación que puebla de imágenes y símbolos el fondo poético de la decadencia contemporánea?" (157). In fact in *Rubén Darío* Rodó accuses Darío himself of an unhealthy, overly sensual application of classical imagery: "...los héroes del *Palimpsesto*, hacen pensar más bien en aquellos blandos y enamoradizos centauros en que degeneró la enflaquecida posteridad de los monstruos biformes, cuando proscritos por la venganza de Hércules, fueron guiados por Neptuno a la isla en que las sirenas tendían sus redes de voluptuosidad" (158).

The possibility of such effeminate, enervating voluptuousness is deliberately purged from the pedagogical setting of *Ariel*. In *Ariel* the socio-cultural and institutional basis for the Hellenic revival is the formation and propagation of morally, socially, intellectually and sentimentally instructive relationships between male youth and an older male mentor. In the ancient Greek model this relationship served to introduce the youth to the many facets of his economic, cultural and sexual position in the social hierarchy; as Eve Kosofsky Sedgwick affirms:

> Thus the love relationship, while temporarily oppressive to the object, had a strongly educational function; Dover quotes Pausanias in Plato's *Symposium* as saying 'that it would be right for him [the boy] to perform any service for one who improves him in mind and character.' Along with its erotic component then, this was a bond of mentorship; the boys were apprentices in the ways and virtues of Athenian citizenship, whose privileges they inherited. (*Between Men* 4)

The erotic and/or homosexual basis of this relationship in the Hellenic tradition, which is expressed in one of *Ariel*'s most influential sources, Plato's *Symposium*, was repressed, purged and, at times, contradictorily underlined by nineteenth-century hellenists both in Europe and Latin America. Moreover, this repressive disassociation between the sensual and the ideal was written into the his-

torical understanding of the Classical period itself and proposed as
the very proof of its humanist integration (Sedgwick, *Epistemology*
138).

In Latin America the contradictory nature of the Hellenic revival of the nineteenth century manifested other functions and conflicts specific to the region's colonial, post and neo-colonial circumstances. In discursive terms the appeal of the Hellenic revival can
be partially explained by the predominance of the European discourses of modernity and the state among large segments of the
Latin American socio-cultural elite. European thinkers of considerable influence in Latin America, such as Ernest Renan and Hippolyte Taine, championed the Greek model in their work. Moreover, as Rafael Gutiérrez Girardot has affirmed, the very foundations of nineteenth century German idealism which linked aesthetics, historiography and the modern state in a shared discourse was
founded on the appreciation of the ancient Greek city-state and its
models for citizenship and cultural development; Gutiérrez Girardot states:

> Ese mundo del hombre íntegro pertenece al pasado, fue el de la
> imagen ideal de Grecia que se había formado desde Winckel-
> mann y a cuyo engrandecimiento contribuyeron además de
> Goethe y Herder, su amigo Hölderlin y el mismo Hegel, quien al
> mirarla con la nostalgia de lo que desapareció dijo, en medio de
> sus complicados análisis de la 'prosa del mundo presente': 'No
> puede haber ni habrá algo más bello'. (39)

Another concept which further anchored the Latin American
intelligentsia in the Hellenic revival was the belief that ancient
Greece was, allegorically speaking, the innocent and youthful period of Western civilization and culture. This anthropomorphic vision of history constructed social, economic, political and cultural
processes in terms of the male body. Greece was projected as the
adolescence of this body and spirit. The conceptualization of Classical civilization and culture in corporal terms aligns the idealist position with the organicist paradigm of bodily, and by extension, social health or illness. Human history since the time of antiquity is
constructed as a healthy or degenerative process of species evolution in spiritual and physical terms according to the ideological and
material conditions of their contemporary setting. This complemen-

tary functioning of a hellenized ideal and an organicist model of national health helps to deconstruct the nineteenth-century binary opposition between spirit/idea and body/matter as well as to challenge the academic critical discourses which separate nineteenth-century idealism and positivism.

For Europe the Hellenic revival had something of a nostalgic aura, a sense of loss or of a necessary return to purity and regeneration. In Latin America, however, this concept of youth coincided with the foundational myth of the unspoiled youth of the lands and peoples of the "New World." In this sense Latin American thinkers could proclaim their societies, cultures and nations to be doubly situated in a state of youth, subsuming both scientific geographical-geological and foundational discourses of the discovery of the New World and the cultural anthropomorphism of the Hellenic model.

Certainly not all Latin American intellectuals of the period were equally enthusiastic about the Hellenic vision of Latin American culture and society. Many felt that it was a direct rejection of the region's own ancient civilizations, such as the Inca or the Aztec, in servile imitation of eurocentric models. This point of view would be found in the indigenist vision of José Carlos Mariátegui or in the stridently pan-Americanist works of José Martí, who in "Nuestra América" offered the following reflection on Hispanic Hellenism: "La historia de América, de los incas acá, ha de enseñarse al dedillo, aunque no se enseñe la de los arcontes de Grecia. Nuestra Grecia es preferible a la Grecia que no es nuestra" (40). From a different political perspective and historical conjunction – that of the emerging Latin American neo-conservatism of the post sixties – there is Carlos Rangel's parodic synopsis of Rodó's affinity with ancient Greece: "Traducción: están reuniendo todo el dinero del mundo en Wall Street, y nos dieron una paliza en Manila y Santiago de Cuba, pero nosotros somos Atenas y *eternos*, y ellos Fenicia y Esparta combinadas, *efímeros*" (95).

Perhaps unwittingly, this neo-conservative ridicule of Rodó's Athenian cultural imagery holds a kernel of truth. There was a contemporary historical impetus for Rodó's Hellenism which transcended the critique of mere eurocentrism. The two-fold threat of Anglo-Saxon imperialism and utilitarianism, along with the menace of cultural infection and imitation, what Rodó's diagnosed as "nordomanía," threatened to "delatinize" *Latin* America:

Es así como la visión de una América *deslatinizada* por propia
voluntad, sin la extorsión de la conquista, y regenerada luego a
imagen y semejanza del arquetipo del Norte... Tenemos nuestra
nordomanía. Es necesario oponerle los límites que la razón y el
sentimiento señalan de consuno. (35)

In response to this threat a new yet nostalgic and politically dis-
armed fraternity arose among certain sectors of the Latin American
and Spanish intelligentsia who sought to protect the cultural identity of "latinidad" from the onslaught of Anglo-Saxon materialism
and intervention,[23] an alliance Juan Durán Luzio has explained in
the following way: "La presencia de una amenaza común reactiva
los lazos entre la Península y las naciones hispánicas de este lado
del Atlántico; el *big stick* se blandía desde Washington tanto a la
una como a las otras" (113).

In Latin America Rodó and the subsequent *arielists* like Francisco García Calderón and Justo Sierra asserted a Latin spirit which
was culturally transmitted through a Latin model of education.
Hence the importance of the pedagogic setting or pretext of *Ariel*.
As Roberto González Echevarría has pointed out in *The Voice of
the Masters: Writing and Authority in Modern Latin America*, the
text of *Ariel* is an educational performance of the humanistic tradition which Rodó sought to reinforce in Latin America. The figure
of the pedagogue, in the text Prospero as the persona of Rodó,
grounds Hispanic culture and identity in a classically dialogical and
rhetorical essayistic form which imparts the archetypical profundity
of the Classical tradition to a Latin American cultural identity.

In this sense *Ariel* helped to inspire the "ateneísta" movement
and the foundation of cultural "ateneos de la juventud" throughout
Latin America. This classical model of Greco-Latin integralist humanism went on to inform the work of the founders of modern
twentieth-century Latin American literary criticism such as Pedro
Henríquez Ureña, who posited a masculine, pedagogically oriented,
Latin cultural identity for Latin America in such essays as "La cul-

---

[23] In Spain thinkers such as Ganivet, Unamuno, Rafael de Altamira, Juan Valera
and Leopoldo Alas (Clarín) either wrote about a pan-Latin culture or directly participated in scholarly fraternal or paternal relationships with the Latin American intelligentsia. For a brief discussion of the Spanish reception and promotion of *Ariel*
see Carlos Real de Azúa's prologue to *Ariel*. Ángel Rama, ed. (Caracas: Biblioteca
Ayacucho, 1976), XXIII.

tura de las humanidades." This humanist Hispanism, as a profession, was contradictorily founded on a critique of the same processes of specialization and the compartamentalization of knowledge which accompanied the modernization of the state and its cultural and educational institutions. [24]

Thus the classical Greek model was not merely (although in some cases it may have been) an elitist form of cultural escapism, but a philological establishment of origins in which the Hellenic civilization served as the legitimizing basis of Latin and Hispanic culture. Moreover, considering the classically and rhetorically based curriculum of the majority of Latin American universities in the nineteenth century, it is not surprising that the Hellenic model should have held some appeal, as it did for Europeans of the period. But unlike the European reception and acceptance of the Hellenic tradition, the Latin American reading of the classical model was fraught with postcolonial tensions. Throughout the colonized regions of world the canonical literature and culture of the hegemonic powers was taught to the partial or complete exclusion of autochthonous or regional cultures. In this way the hegemonic culture became an oppressive standard of measurement which was inscribed into the aesthetic national consciousness of the colonized peoples. Considered from this perspective, Rodó's *Ariel* takes on the monumental task of disarming and appropriating what could be described as the most important tenet of the eurocentric theory of universal cultural value, namely, the Classical tradition. This bold seizure of the Classical tradition becomes doubly ambitious if we consider that it is situated in a text which appropriates another cultural cornerstone of European hegemony in the New World, Shakespeare's *The Tempest*. [25]

---

[24] For an insightful discussion of this process see Julio Ramos, "Masa, Cultura, Latinoamericanismo," in *Desencuentros de la modernidad en América Latina* (Mexico: Fondo de Cultura Económica, 1989), 202-228.

[25] In this light Rob Nixon's assertion about Caribbean re-writings of *The Tempest* would also hold true for Rodó. Nixon states in "Caribbean and African Appropriations of *The Tempest*":

> In discussions of value, Shakespeare is, of course, invariably treated as a special case, having come to serve as something like the gold standard of literature. For the English he is as much an institution as an industry as a corpus of texts: a touchstone of national identity, a lure for tourists, an exportable commodity, and one of the securest forms of cultural capital around. But the weight of Shakespeare's ascribed authority was felt dif-

HEALTHY INTROSPECTION VS SICKLY SELF-ABSORPTION

In *Ariel* the assertion that Latin America was the torch-bearer of Greco-Roman civilization and culture fits squarely into the medical paradigm of national regeneration. Both in general metaphysical terms and in specific textual images Rodó associates ancient Greece with male adolescence, thereby inscribing Hellenic idealism into the health or sickness of the masculine body. By linking Latin America to ancient Greece, Rodó appropriated Hegel's assertion that Hellenic civilization represented the adolescence of the world spirit, thereby ascribing agency to Latin America in the development of what Hegel termed "the Idea." Therefore, in both philosophical and physiological terms, Rodó prescribes youth and ancient Greece as a kind of spiritual-national tonic for cultural regeneration.

This tonic, Rodó affirms, is readily available within Latin America's youth and only requires the spiritual faith and confidence in itself in order to activate its dynamic properties. Here Rodó is introducing a central concept in his spiritual-somatic program of regeneration, namely, that spiritual ideals can be transformed into vital force or energy. This notion comes, in large measure, from Rodó's interest in the work of Fouillée and his concept of the "idée-force," a concept which, as we have already seen, was also of considerable importance to the Spaniard Ganivet.[26]

Very early in his final lecture, Prospero, the fictional teacher of *Ariel*'s literary pretext, informs his students that this potential life-force is already within them and only awaits their own self-belief and self-love in order to become energized:

> ...debéis empezar por reconocer un primer objeto de fe, en vosotros mismos. La juventud que vivís es una fuerza de cuya

---

ferently in the colonies. What was for the English a source of pride and a confirmation of their civilization, for colonial subjects often became a chastening yardstick of their "backwardness." The exhortation to master Shakespeare was instrumental in showing up non-European "inferiority," for theirs would be the flawed mastery of those culturally remote from Shakespeare's stock. (560)

[26] Gordon Brotherston, in the introduction to his edition of *Ariel*, refers to the influence of Fouillée's *L'idée moderne du droit* on Rodó.

aplicación sois los obreros y un tesoro de cuya inversión sois res-
ponsables. Amad ese tesoro y esa fuerza; haced que el altivo
sentimiento de su posesión permanezca ardiente y eficaz en
vosotros. (2-3)

Jaime Concha has underlined the tautological nature of Prospero's
assertion that youth is an act of faith, that "La juventud es fe en la
juventud,..." (125). Yet although the triggering of this healing energy is introspective in nature, the teacher Prospero-Rodó is also informing the students that this energy has an extra-personal or collective function. He tells them that they are "responsible" for the
investment of this social resource, a responsibility he will elaborate
upon at length throughout the essay.

Rodó equates this "treasure" of youth with "light," "love," and
"energy" which revitalize the "proceso evolutivo de las sociedades"
(4). These spiritual and physical forces constitute the therapeutic
energy of Latin American youth. Prospero directly interrelates the
regenerative qualities of his student audience's youth with those of
ancient Greece when he offers this ancient civilization as the
archetypal manifestation of ageless vitality:

> Hubo una vez en que los atributos de la juventud humana se
> hicieron, más que en ninguna otra, los atributos de un pueblo,
> los caracteres de una civilización, y en que un soplo de adoles-
> cencia encantadora pasó rozando la frente serena de una raza.
> Cuando Grecia nació, los dioses le regalaron el secreto de su ju-
> ventud inextinguible. Grecia es el alma joven. (4)

In this passage about Greece's eternal youth the regenerative
power of adolescence is ascribed the divine quality of a breath of
air, "un soplo de adolescencia encantadora," which recalls the scientific associations of revitalizing fresh air and ventilation connoted
by the aerist figure of Ariel. Shortly thereafter, Rodó elaborates on
the restorative powers of youth, connecting spiritually invigorating
properties to physically activating forces: "Las prendas del espíritu
joven –el entusiasmo y la esperanza– corresponden en las armonías
de la historia y la naturaleza, al movimiento de la luz" (5). This alliance between pagan-Christian idealism, the spiritual elixirs of "en-
thusiasm" and "hope," together with the kinetically physical properties of "the movement of light," infuse Rodó's idealism with a

dose of scientific materialism that is a constant in the text. The conversion of spiritual energy into mechanical energy reiterates the transformation of ideas into force, the formula of Fouillée's "idéeforce."

Yet, as Rodó forewarns with his exhortation regarding youth's responsibility, this force can be dishonored, poorly spent and dissipated. The loss is equally individual and social because the rejuvenating benefits squandered by the individual cannot be enjoyed by society at large. Prospero reminds the students of the dangers involved: "Sed, pues, conscientes poseedores de la fuerza bendita que lleváis dentro de vosotros mismos. No creáis, sin embargo, que ella está extenta de malograrse y desvanecerse, como un impulso sin objeto en la realidad" (5). Nature, "De la Naturaleza es la dávida del precioso tesoro...," is the source of this energy and transgressions against nature result in sterile waste.

Such language concerning the retention of youthful male energy and the potential danger of its loss through infertile expenditure conjures up the nineteenth-century medical discourse concerning physical, spiritual and psychological dissipation through the promiscuous exercise of sexual activity we have already noted in Ganivet. Situated in the chaste male company of the classroom whose muse is Ariel – the manifestation of virtuous triumph over the earth, femininity, sexuality, in short, over Caliban – the analogy between male youth's internal life-force and semen acquires greater force. In fact, Rodó provides a literary case-study of self-inflicted, overly sensual, promiscuous enervation as a negative example of the possibility of premature degeneration.

The novel by "un escritor sagaz" which Rodó holds up as a negative mirror is Joris-Karl Huysmans' *À Rebours* (1884). This influential fin-de-siècle novel follows the life of an extremely dissolute, effete, sickly, young aristocrat, Des Esseintes, as he plumbs the depths of feverish, sensual and languid self-indulgence. The dissolute nature of Des Esseintes' aesthetic reverie was not lost on contemporary theorists of cultural enervation such as Max Nordau who affirmed that: "The Duke Jean des Esseintes is physically an anaemic and nervous man of weak constitution, the inheritor of all the vices and all the degeneracies of an exhausted race" (302).

In the context of *Ariel*, *À Rebours* underlines the sickly side of the cultural model of aesthetic self-development, a model which Rodó nervously shares. The character of Des Esseintes' is associated with the "unnatural vices" of "self-abuse": masturbation and homosexuality. Rodó presents this novel to his students as a seductively dangerous account of the threat of youthful degeneration:

> ... –esa inmensa superficie especular donde se refleja toda entera la imagen de la vida en los últimos vertiginosos cien años– la psicología, los estados de alma de la juventud, tales como ellos han sido en las generaciones que van desde los días de René hasta los que han visto pasar a Des Esseintes. Su análisis comprobaba una progresiva disminución de *juventud interior* y de energía, en la serie de personajes representativos que se inicia con los héroes, enfermos, pero a menudo viriles y siempre intensos de pasión, de los románticos, y termina con los enervados de voluntad y corazón en quienes se reflejan tan desconsoladoras manifestaciones del espíritu como la del protagonista de *A Rebours* o la del Robert Greslou de *Le Disciple*. (6)

Unlike the external threat of cultural, spiritual and bodily infection and enervation personified in the symbol of Caliban and internalized in Latin America as "nordomanía," the degenerative threat to Latin American health posed by the model of Huysman's Des Esseintes is internal to Rodó's cultural model of introspective cultural development. Des Esseintes' exaggeration of inward cultivation becomes a wanton life of unmanly self-indulgence which fruitlessly expends male youth in decadent pastimes. Rodó's instructive synopsis of the novel reinforces the need for masculine self-control within the introspective project of national regeneration.

Rodó's appraisal of *À Rebours* is at once reverent yet distant; this tale of youthful decline is an instructive and entertaining place to visit but he would not want to live there. The admiring yet condemning allusion to Huysmans is directed as much at himself and his fellow *modernistas* as it is at his vulnerable students. It is generally understood that the literature of European decadence was very influential in turn-of-the-century Latin American literature. But this interest was not without conflicts nor anxiety, inasmuch as Latin American intellectuals seeking to establish an aesthetics for their emerging nations were not enthusiastic about offering a model in which Latin Americans would identify with an effeminate, sensual and sickly protagonist, poetics or narrative. On the contrary, *Ariel*, like the other essays under discussion in this study were written within a scientific and medical paradigm which classified these qualities as being the sources of national debility and weakness.

It was out of this anxiety concerning the sickly influence of French decadent literature that Rodó wrote *Rubén Darío* (1899), a critical appraisal of Rubén Darío's poetry in which he categorically stated that: "Indudablemente, Rubén Darío no es el poeta de América" (137). In fact Rodó's *Rubén Darío* anticipates many of the aesthetic, discursive and thematic structures of *Ariel*, and, in what is of importance for this current study, explicitly ties them into theories of national degeneration and/or regeneration. According to Rodó's admiring yet censorious evaluation, Darío's poetry inscribed excessively ornamental, sensual, and effeminate language and imagery into the Latin American consciousness. Rodó found this to be particularly egregious given the youthful vulnerability of Latin American literature and identity. Rodó unhesitatingly described these alleged traits as symptoms of potential illness: "¿No crees tú que tal concepción de la poesía encierra un grave peligro, un peligro mortal, para esa arte divina, puesto que, a fin de hacerla 'enfermar de selección' se limita a la luz, el aire, el jugo de tierra?" (144). Here what Rodó had earlier described as an unhealthy and claustrophobic "parnasianismo extendido al mundo interior" specifically excludes the healing agents of light and air which are so fundamental to *Ariel*.

What Rodó can safely admit to admiring in the works of French decadence is their critique of modernization. This critique manifests itself in *Ariel* through what Rodó calls a sensibility of "*extrañeza, del espíritu*," an ambivalent term which suggests both a circumstantial or social estrangement and a constitutional or characterological strangeness. While Rodó can, in good conscience, identify with the notion of social alienation implied by "*extrañeza*," he anxiously disassociates himself from the characterological oddness it implies. In doing so Rodó expresses his phobia regarding the degenerate, effeminate or homosexual nature of the elitist rejection of modernity, a rejection which he regards as sickly: "no es necesario aproximarse al parnasianismo de estirpe delicada y enferma, a quien un aristocrático desdén de lo presente llevó a la reclusión en lo pasado" (29).

The error of Darío was to conceive of his Latin American poetry in affinity with the work of the French symbolist Verlaine. Rodó characterizes the latter as the very model of the degenerate youth

whose mixture of "barbarie y de bizantinismo, de infancia y de ca-
ducidad, de perversión y de ternura..." (164) culminates in the
"*Crimen amoris* verleniano" (165). Not only does Rodó rely here
upon metaphorically cloaked models of degeneracy theory to de-
nounce the threat of "decadent" literature and behaviors, he also
cites one of clinical degeneracy theory's most ardent exponents,
Max Nordau, who made theories of neurological degeneration the
basis for his critique of literature in his widely read *Degeneration*
(1892). In *Rubén Darío* Rodó cites Nordau while contemplating the
qualities of "los Raros" which make them "strange": "Y la cuestión
no debe parecerle enteramente trivial, si considera que el talento de
encontrar títulos buenos es el único que ha querido reconocer Max
Nordau a los oficiantes de las nuevas capillas literarias, esos clientes
'malgré eux' de su clínica" (168).[27]

In *Ariel* the cautionary counter-example of Des Esseintes and
the perils of French decadence does not, however, completely allay
Rodó's anxiety concerning the potential for the internal corruption
of youth within his own introspective program for cultural self-development. The figure of the degenerate youth Des Esseintes together with a certain phobia concerning the homosexual overtones
of the Platonic model of masculine self and group cultivation combine to haunt Rodó throughout *Ariel*. Such fears are openly expressed in rhetorical questions concerning the possibility of adolescent degeneration or aboulia. Immediately after discussing Huysmans Rodó wonders whether the potential for Platonic regeneration inspired by adolescent male muses is still possible now that
the Spring-like innocence of the Hellenic period of youth is over:

> ¿no nos será lícito, a lo menos, soñar con la aparición de genera-
> ciones humanas que devuelvan a la vida un sentido ideal, un
> grande entusiasmo; en las que sea un poder el sentimiento, en las
> que una vigorosa resurrección de las energías de la voluntad
> ahuyente, con heroico clamor, del fondo de las almas, todas las
> cobardías morales que se nutren a los pechos de la decepción y

---

[27] It is interesting to note that Darío himself launched a counter-attack against
Nordau and neuropathological literary criticism in general in an ongoing exchange
in *La Nación*. In his reply "Al Dr. Nordau" Darío states: "En verdad, Max Nordau
no deja un solo nombre, entre todos los escritores y artistas contemporáneos de la
aristocracia intelectual, al lado del cual no escriba la correspondiente clasificación
diagnóstica: 'imbécil', 'idiota', 'degenerado', 'loco peligroso'". See "Max Nordau,"
Rubén Darío. Obras Completas, vol. 2 (Madrid: Afrodisio Aguado, 1950-53), 451.

de la duda? ¿Será de nuevo la juventud una realidad de la vida
colectiva, como lo es de la vida individual? (6)

Here Rodó expresses doubt concerning Latin American youth's
ability to stimulate the weakened state of the region's health. It is a
decidedly Fouillée-inspired formulation of spirit transfigured into
therapeutic energy and action in which the power of "sentimiento"
engenders a "resurrección" of energy and volition. Answering his
own question, Rodó optimistically states that such apparently
pathological states of doubt are but a fleeting aberration of youthful
introspection inherent to the self-searching faith and energy of
youth: "Tal es la pregunta que me inquieta mirándoos. Vuestras
primeras páginas, las confesiones que nos habéis hecho hasta ahora
de vuestro mundo íntimo, hablan de indecisión y de estupor a
menudo; nunca de enervación, ni de un definitivo quebranto de la
voluntad" (7). This question-answer series reproduces the ambiguity concerning the medical discourse of regeneration at play in the
text. On the one hand Latin America and its youth are in need of a
regeneration or "resurrección" of energy and will; on the other
hand Rodó denies that this need reflects a pathological state, af-
firming that it is more a byproduct of youth itself and the "juventud
de los pueblos" than constitutional illness. Yet it is Rodó who repeatedly brings up the issue and terminology of enervation, obsessively invoking that which he wishes to deny, such as in the following passage about adolescent aboulia: "Cuando el dolor enerva;
cuando el dolor es la irresistible pendiente que conduce al marasmo
o el consejero pérfido que mueve a la abdicación de la voluntad, la
filosofía que le lleva en sus entrañas es cosa indigna de almas
jóvenes" (8).

Returning to his original tautological definition of youth, Rodó
affirms that this kind of degeneration can either be cured or avoided through faith in oneself and the future: "La fe en el porvenir, la
confianza en la eficacia del esfuerzo humano, son el antecedente
necesario de toda acción enérgica y de todo propósito fecundo" (8).
But he remains uncertain about the purity of youthful energy when
turned inward on itself. This ongoing anxiety reflects the convergence of two developments of the late nineteenth century, one
socio-historical, the other medical.

The socio-historical process I am referring to is the very *introspective* nature of Rodó's program for national rejuvenation. The

exhortation to youth that they will discover their individually and socially revitalizing life-force when they look inward and believe in themselves is not a concept exclusive to Rodó. Rather, it constitutes part of a larger social and psychological response to modernity whose complexity can only be generally outlined in the context of this study.

The nineteenth century witnessed the manifold processes of the technological modernization of labor and the massification and commercialization of social relations and culture. As we have seen in the case of Ganivet, in response to these alienating processes nineteenth-century intellectuals rallied around the concept of spiritual human values which were felt to be antithetical to the massive rationalization of the period. Such spiritual values were said to be found within the self or individual, initiating a divisive break between the true inner core of the individual and the historical processes and social practices which constitute a social subject. But the perception of this break paradoxically demonstrated the continuing ties between nineteenth-century intellectuals and artists and their social environment for, as Gutiérrez Girardot has pointed out:

> Negación del presente y evasión a otros mundos: estas son las características del artista en la moderna sociedad burguesa. Pero ella no significa, como se suele insistir, que el artista huye de la realidad. Por paradójico que parezca, el artista no hace otra cosa que vivir dentro de esta realidad que detesta, la del hombre burgués, que también huye de la realidad y se refugia, como observó Benjamin, en su '*intérieur*'... (56)

The Latin American experience of this perceived opposition between interior and exterior reality differed from the European case in terms of quantity and quality. Certainly the effects and consequences of transnational capitalist economic development and commerce had a considerable impact on economic, social and cultural life in Latin America. In the country of Rodó, the penetration of British capital and influence at the end of the nineteenth century, subsequently replaced by North American interests in the early twentieth century, accelerated the transformation of Uruguay from a pre-capitalist economy into a dependent component of an international market organized according to the international division of labor (Achugar 30). But "modernization" also produced a psychological sensibility of social rupture for segments of the cultural and economic elites of the more developed urban centers like Montevideo. Whether this sense of disempowerment engendered by modernization manifested itself in intellectual psycho-cultural introspection or political resistance, it certainly did not, as Hugo Achugar has stressed, go unnoticed: "Dicho proceso [modernization] no se realiza, sin embargo, sin luchas ni conflictos, ya que se efectúa en una realidad determinada histórica y socialmente que, lejos de funcionar como un mero marco pasivo de referencia, dialécticamente impulsará o resistirá dicho proceso" (Achugar 30).

However, the introduction and consolidation of the rationalizing technological and financial processes of liberal modernization was uneven and fragmented in Latin America, leading to different regional or even national experiences. As Ángel Rama asserts: "Este ingreso no es parejo en toda la comarca hispanoparlante, ni tiene la misma intensidad en sus diversas zonas, como ya lo anotara Henríquez Ureña, viéndolo bajo el ángulo de la prosperidad" (27).

As a consequence of this fragmented and uneven character of modernization in Latin America, the site of its experience was in a sense more discursively centered. This notion squares with the important role that literature has played in the foundation of Latin American nations and identities. In effect, the sphere of literature and literary values comes into opposition to rationalization, serving thus as an alternative organizing principle pitting interior against exterior experience. Julio Ramos has described this split in the following way:

> Entre la máquina y la literatura, entonces media la *antítesis*. Pero esa representación de la tecnología, según veremos, se encuentra profundamente ideologizada. La antítesis es un mecanismo de orden, de organización de una realidad compleja, contradictoria. La *figura* facilita la formulación de un afuera, lugar de máquina amenazante, en cuyo reverso se constituye un adentro, *reino interior* en que se consolida y adquiere especificidad la literatura y otras zonas de producción estética. (158)

The other development which further grounds Rodó's anxiety about youthful introspection in a larger socio-historical context is the increasing medical attention that degeneracy theorists and psychologists paid to infantile sexuality. This preoccupation characterized the work of Bénedict-Augustin Morel, whose *Traité des dégénérescences* (1857) was one of the foundational texts of degeneracy theory. Morel theorized the syndrome of *dementia praecox* which shifted the association of degeneration away from the elderly to the young (Carlson 129). Once again, premature enervation was linked to masturbation and other unwarranted exercises of youthful sexuality. Competing Romantic theories of the purity of children could not dislodge this association and, as Sander Gilman states, "Nevertheless the concept of degeneracy remained linked to childhood, to illness, and to childhood sexuality" ("Sexology" 80).

These conflicting notions of physical and spiritual purity of youth vs. its inherently degenerative qualities are evident throughout the history, from pre-Shakespearean sources through Rodó, of the Prospero-Ariel-Caliban triangle. Both Ariel and Caliban are in a sense Prospero's children, or at least wards. Ariel is the pure, innocent, asexual youth free from bodily passions, while Caliban is the lecherous "native," who lusts after his master's daughter Miranda. Such dichotomous views of youth are situated in the discursive constructions of the indigenous inhabitants of the New World which Shakespeare encompassed in *The Tempest*.

The Historical Roots of Ariel and Caliban as Symbols of Health and Disease

Both as an image and as an ideal, Ariel is a body without organs other than the brain. According to Rodó it is this cerebral power and beauty which will regenerate Latin America. Caliban, on the other hand, until his "revision" by authors such as Roberto Fernández Retamar, is the very manifestation of the New World's alleged anatomical, aesthetic and spiritual inferiority. As Shakespeare and his precursors constructed him, Caliban is a monster, a half-man, half-beast curiosity to be exploited for financial gain as Trinculo states in *The Tempest*:

> A strange fish! Were I in England now (as once I was), and had but this fish painted, not a holiday fool there but would give a piece of silver: there would this monster make a man; any strange beast there makes a man: when they will not give a doit to relive a lame beggar, they will lay out ten to see a dead Indian. Legg'd

like a man! and his fins like arms! Warm, o' my troth! I do now let loose my opinion, hold it no longer; this is no fish but an islander... (act II, scene II)

Here Shakespeare expresses many of the notions which characterize the hegemonic Western visions of conquered peoples, an ideology of subjugation which acquired scientific legitimacy in the eighteenth and nineteenth centuries. Specifically, the passage outlines the claims soon to be empirically "confirmed" that colonialized peoples are unhygienic, smelly, unhealthy and non-evolved creatures suited only to serving the superior races. The proto-evolutionary attention to the species differentiation between upright bipeds ("Legg'd like a man") and lower species, together with confusion over appendage development ("his fins like arms") is resolved by the logical conclusion that this is a sub-species different from both: "this is no fish but an islander."

Moreover, unlike Ariel, Caliban is associated with the damp earth and darkness of his cave dwelling. As opposed to Ariel's masculine, dry, healing light he embodies a feminine, wet, decaying darkness. In *Ariel*, Rodó associates the masses with this feminine calibanesque darkness: they live "envuelto en una sombra" (10); they constitute a degenerate "civilización que vivió para tejerse un sudario y para edificar los sepulcros: la sombra de un compás teniéndose sobre la esterilidad de la arena" (5); they are a "masa indiferente y oscura" (59) whose transitory power is no more than "una noche de sueño en la existencia de la humanidad" (51).

In *The Tempest* the swampy, lustful, deformed and biologically inferior figure of Caliban is directly associated with disease. His ailment is both congenital and environmental, posing a threat to those around him. Prospero condemns his slave as an incurable degenerate who suffers from a physical and mental *dementia praecox*: "A devil, a born devil, on whose nature nurture can never stick; on whom my pains, humanely taken, all, all lost, quite lost: And as with age, his body uglier grows, so his mind cankers..." (act IV, scene I). Caliban himself is aware of his alleged association with illness and seeks to appropriate this debility in order to infect his master and tormentor, Prospero, with a spell of disease conjured from the sickly surroundings of the island: "All the infections that the sun sucks up from bogs, fens, flats, on Prospero fall, and make him by inch-meal a disease!" (act II, scene II).

In *Ariel*, Rodó does little to dispel the aura of biological and psychological pathology surrounding the figure of Caliban. While Rodó deflects some of the force of the association onto what he considers the degenerate materialism of the United States, this does not fully dislodge Caliban's identification with internal Latin American corruption. As I previously noted, the externalization of Caliban had an internally complementary and debilitating reverberation in the disorder of "nordomanía."

Of greater significance is the fact that Rodó retained the sexually degenerate characterization of Caliban, which is inextricably tied into the gendered, biological denigration of indigenous populations. On the first page of *Ariel*, immediately following a Darwinist, and therefore inherently bio-racial appraisal of Ariel's superiority, Caliban is stereotypically impugned the degenerative sensuality of the non-white races; "...Calibán, símbolo de sensualidad y de torpeza..." This racial construction of Caliban is rephrased throughout the text in discussions linking calibanesque irrationality and uncontrollable sexuality, for example the following passage: "Los hombres y los pueblos trabajan, en el sentido de Fouillée, bajo la inspiración de las ideas, como los irracionales bajo la inspiración de los instintos..." (56). The euphemism "irracionales" could apply equally to women, criminals, sexual deviants, children, the "inferior races" or all of the above.

The suggestion of Caliban's ethnic and sexual enervation is also indicated by intimations of sexual deviancy within democracy. Sexual, racial and political perversion is rendered as bestiality, recalling the Shakespearean Caliban's monstrous desire to "mate" with Miranda and populate the island with a cross-breed sub-species of "Calibans." Rodó refers to egalitarian democracy as a "*zoocracia*" where "La Tatiana de Shakespeare, poniendo un beso en la cabeza asinina, podría ser el emblema de la Libertad que ortorga su amor a los mediocres. ¡Jamás, por medio de una conquista más fecunda podrá llegarse a un resultado más fatal!" (28). This sexually charged and comical depiction of miscegenation and social mobility within democracy proves to be quite "racy" for the supposedly spiritually aloof Rodó.

Rodó's vision of the figure of Caliban also borrows from Ernest Renan's reactionary and racist version of *The Tempest*, *Caliban*, *suite de La Tempête* (1878). In this work Renan condemns the Commune of 1870 as the product of a congenitally and sexually degen-

erate working class which Rodó calls the "entronización de Calibán" (24). Yet Rodó, following Fouillée, was unsettled by the cyn-
ical·triumph of the degenerate Caliban of Renan's drama and wrote
Ariel in order to restore Ariel as a symbol of regeneration. [28] Rodó's
reference to the defeat of Ariel in Renan's work vindicates the symbol's eternal powers of regeneration. The image crafted by Rodó
gives Ariel a phoenix-like aura which enables the spirit to repeatedly rise from the ashes and other dejecta. The following passage once
again borrows from the discourse of biological, racial and sexual
degeneracy ascribed to the non-white inhabitants of Latin America:

> Vencido una y mil veces por la indomable rebelión de Calibán,
> proscrito por la barbarie vencedora, asfixiado en el humo de las
> batallas, manchadas las alas transparentes al rozar el "eterno es-
> tercolero de Job", Ariel resurge inmortalmente, Ariel recobra su
> juventud y su hermosura, y acude ágil, como al mandato de
> Próspero, al llamado de cuantos le amen en la realidad. (58)

The concept of an uncontrollable and unjust national uprising
led by supposedly "inferior" elements of society, the Calibans and
their "barbarie vencedora," clearly reproduces the nineteenth-century Latin American discourse of civilization versus racial, sexual and
political barbarism established in such canonical texts as Sarmiento's *Facundo: civilización y barbarie*. Moreover, this passage reiterates the binary oppositions of health-illness and spirit-body clus-
tered around the figures of Ariel and Caliban. Ariel is the immortal,
organ-less body of immaterial transparent wings forever rising to
youthful regeneration. Caliban, on the other hand, is associated
with the colon and excrement, an undeniable, essential but ideologically repudiated product of the body. The psychological aversion
to excrement expressed social suspicion felt by the middle class for
convicts, prostitutes, the insane, non-aryans, homosexuals and the
working class (Corbin 145). The excremental aura of these
marginalized groups was attributed, in an interrelated manner, to
their physiognomical constitution, the terms of their confinement,
the filth of their employment – both circumstantial, as in the case of
tanners, rag-pickers etc., and moral, such as prostitutes, and their

---

[28] For a discussion of the triangle between Renan, Fouillée and Rodó, see
Brotherston's introduction to his edition of *Ariel*, 2-6.

sexual practices. All of these groups were associated with decay and illness and as such posed a threat to public or national health.

In *Ariel*, this connection between excrement, illness and racial inferiority is represented in the reference to the biblical figure of Job. The association between Job and excrement was not unique to Rodó (Corbin 145). Job became the symbolic embodiment of the dung-man whose putrefied exhalations threatened the collective health. In *Ariel*, Caliban, "el eterno estercolero de Job," literally soils Ariel's wings, ("manchadas las alas") with his infectious excrement. This provocative scatological construction of Caliban consolidates the racial, sexual and social components of his congenital degeneracy.

Perhaps the most concentrated example of Rodó's unresolved tension in *Ariel* concerning the healthy innocence or corruptible vulnerability of youth centers around the didactic tale he concocts about an Oriental king. Seemingly unsatisfied that the negative example of Huysmans' Des Esseintes has sufficiently inoculated his students, Prospero relates the allegorical fable of a king who cultivated his internal spiritual garden. It is in effect an example of what Rodó termed the "estética de la conducta," a problematic notion of psychological harmony based on an analogy between aesthetic beauty and social organization (Brotherston 8).

Importantly, the fable is prefaced with the following injunctions about the dangers of self-absorption: "No entreguéis nunca a la utilidad o a la pasión, sino una parte de vosotros. Aun dentro de la esclavitud material, hay la posibilidad de salvar la libertad interior: la de la razón y el sentimiento" (12). Once again, this cautionary remark equates sensuality, "pasión," with the vulgarity of materialism, "utilidad." Nevertheless this allegedly instructive tale betrays Rodó's own attachments to the narrative of European decadence and orientalism. We consider the sensual description of the king's palace:

> Mercaderes de Ofir, buhoneros de Damasco, cruzaban a toda hora las puertas anchurosas, y ostentaban en competencia, ante las miradas del rey, las telas, las joyas, los perfumes... Los fatigados vientos abandonaban largamente sobre el alcázar real su carga de aromas y armonías. Empinándose desde el vecino mar, como si quisieran ceñirle en un abrazo, le salpicaban las olas con su espuma. Y una libertad paradisial, una inmensa reciprocidad de confianzas, mantenían por dondequiera la animación de una fiesta inextinguible... (13)

The apparent sensuality of this exterior is supposedly offset by the chaste serenity of the palace's interior chamber. As Prospero tells his students "dentro, muy adentro...," a room where the light "llegaba lánguida"; "velaba en ella la castidad del aire dormido." Rodó undercuts the notion of chastity with the sensual images of languor. This ambiguity continues in the paradoxically sensual and chaste description of an olfactory sensation: "En el ambiente flota-ba como una onda indisipable la casta esencia de nenúfar, el per-fume sugeridor del adormecimiento penseroso y de la contem-plación del propio ser." Such a description suggests at once subli-mation and olfactory over-indulgence, a practice highly denounced by nineteenth-century physicians along with other forms of "self-abuse." [29]

The apotheosis of the fable of the king is a dream the king has while lost in self-contemplation within the sanctuary of his exclu-sive inner chamber. In this dream the king envisions himself achiev-ing the ultimate state of internal freedom and harmony:

> En él soñaba, en él se libertaba de la realidad, el rey legendario; en él sus miradas se volvían a lo interior y se bruñían en la me-ditación sus pensamientos como guijas lavadas por la espuma; en él se desplegaban sobre su noble frente las blancas alas de Psiquis... (14)

The description of the dream establishes a concentric system of in-creasingly inward layers of introspection which are situated at once within the chamber, the self and the unconscious. It is noteworthy that the inward trajectory of the story is reproduced by an increas-ing degree of irreality and fantasy. The fact that *Ariel* is itself a fic-tional narrative of exemplary self-constitution is more deeply grounded in spiritual nihilism by this didactic account of a dream which breaks with reality in order to reach the "última Thule" of the soul. The only substantial material presence in this tale is the wafting cloud of perfumed air, which, as González Echevarría as-serts, is a rather ethereal substance for self-constitution: "The con-templation of the self, the constitution of the self, occurs within this

---

[29] On the nineteenth century view that perfume exercised an immoral, un-healthy influence, Alain Corbin states: "The charm of perfumes, the search for 'base sensations,' symptoms of a 'soft, lax' education, increased nervous irritability, led to 'feminism,' and encouraged debauchery" (184).

undifferentiated, transparent, almost non-existent substance in which reflection cannot be true. Here being can be itself, identity is found in chaste indivisibility, in inviolable self-presence" (22).

As the reader (along with Prospero's fictional students) are led deeper into the recesses of the king's spiritual interior, there is an accompanying increase in the alleged purity of the king's reflection which reaches a somewhat rhapsodic state in a spiritual union with the figure of Psyche. On the surface this union is one which speaks of a spiritual purity not entirely unlike that of the mystic poet's bodily descriptions of spiritual union with God. But by the same token, it is possible to challenge the theoretical underpinnings of purity for just such a union. Beyond the fact that the image of Psyche comes to the king in an over-charged moment of self-absorption, indulgence or "abuse," the very image or concept of Psyche and what she connotes is at issue. For in addition to her identification with the human soul, she is also associated, through her connection to Cupid, with love and desire. The classicist Richmond Hathorn has summarized the connotations surrounding Psyche as follows: "*Psyche* means 'soul'; centuries earlier Plato (*Phaedrus* 246, 251-252) had pictured the soul as growing wings and ascending to a higher plane under the influence of Eros." Thus Psyche is not an entirely chaste figure. As a consequence, throughout the ages Psyche has been associated and confused with Pandora: "Like Pandora, with her unmastered curiosity leading to the breaking of a taboo, Psyche could easily be regarded as a pagan Eve, and her story could be allegorized by Christian writers to represent the soul's damnation and salvation" (Hathorn 244-245).

The ambiguity of this fantasized contact with Psyche further challenges the notion of chastity and disinterest within the text. In this sense declarations and avowals of spiritual, asexual detachment cannot be accepted at face value, and the discursive "repression" of sexuality in the text should not be seen as an exclusion of interest in the sexual, but rather as a re-channeling of such interest into another socially or morally legitimate plane. It is in this light that we should consider the tale of the Oriental king, a tale which Rodó qualifies as the "escenario de vuestro reino interior" (14). It is a scene, Rodó adds, that is premised upon the necessity of leisure or "ocio" which he traces back to his de-eroticized version of the Classical tradition. But in *Ariel*, the self-involved, idle and class-inflected nature of this leisure is somewhat muted by Rodó's addition that its languid and sensual character has been corrected by the "moderna creencia en la dignidad del trabajo útil." Yet this is an amendment designed to address sexual anxiety which rings hollow in the larger anti-utilitarian, culturalist context of the text. For the leisure enjoyed by the king retains its self-absorbed, sensual tone.

This ambiguous, if not decadent, leisure realigns Rodó's fictionally therapeutic protagonists, Prospero and the Oriental king, with Huysmans' sickly youth Des Esseintes. All three possess the social privilege of a state of leisure which permits them the luxury of self-contemplation or absorption. What proves to be a much more provocative point of contact for these figures, however, is that in their moments of self-contemplation they fixate upon androgynous, adolescent figures for inspiration and/or renewal. This reliance upon images of sexually ambivalent youth further entwines *Ariel* in conflicting and interrelated theories of the universality, health and/or degeneracy of the nineteenth century's vision of the youthful androgyne.

THE THERAPEUTIC QUALITIES OF THE ANDROGYNOUS ADOLESCENT MALE

In *Ariel*, as noted, there is an implicit association between the figure of Ariel, the symbolic embodiment of reason and spirit, and Psyche, the symbolic personification of the soul. These two beings share many important attributes and functions beyond their connections to spirituality. They are lithe, winged and not yet anatomically mature. This physical immaturity manifests itself through a lack of strongly differentiating sexual, or gender identifying physiognomies. Their youthful androgyny is also intersected by a shared function, that of visionary muse to an older male. In *Ariel*, Psyche inspires the Oriental king while Ariel stimulates Prospero.

Even in its more aesthetic and idealist articulations, Rodó's concept of regenerative ideals, healing beauty and youthful force is tied into the image of an androgynous, winged and immature male body. Moreover, Rodó states that these revitalizing ideals are not spontaneously generated in a void but that they germinate in this body: "Las ideas adquieren alas potentes y veloces, no en el seno de la abstracción, sino en el luminoso y cálido ambiente de la forma" (21). Not only does Rodó connect the ideal to the pubescent, androgynous body, as "encantadoras exterioridades de la naturaleza," but he goes on to situate this idea-body in the evolutionary process. The beauty of these bodies is compared to the biological function, "una función realísima," of beauty in nature which attracts members of a species to one another for reproduction. Thus androgynous male beauty is attributed the evolutionary function of selecting and advancing the species in a process which "han hecho prevalecer, dentro de cada especie, a los seres mejor dotados de hermosura sobre los menos ventajosamente dotados" (22).

This functional and anatomical similarity between Psyche and Ariel points to another point of discursive and philosophical confluence which inscribes Rodó's idealism within the late nineteenth century scientific theories of the inferiority of women and species differentiation. There were many ways of specifying evolution and differentiation within the species of *homo sapiens*. The possible progression or regression of the species could be described in terms of age, race or gender according to the given context of the discussion. Frequently, these categories were interrelated in a complementary fashion which aligned sexual with racial evolution.

In terms of age and gender, human evolution was seen as moving from an original state of universal bisexuality to increasingly differentiated male and female genders. In the *Descent of Man*, Darwin had remarked on the anatomical resemblance between the male and female offspring of humans and other species. This morphological resemblance between the young of both sexes was seen to resemble that of the adult female. This state of undifferentiated resemblance between the young and the female was contrasted to the distinctly "evolved" physiognomy of the adult male (Dijkstra 198). The health of the race was linked to an accelerating pace of biologically determined sexual, social, political and economic differentiation between the two genders. This process initiated progressive as well as regressive evolutionary trends. As women became more "feminine" they became increasingly unable to disassociate themselves from their role in biological reproduction. Biologists, sexologists and psychologists claimed that this role consumed and exhausted their energies, leaving them little vital force to pursue intellectual or spiritual endeavors. Women were biologically locked into a state of nature for the benefit of the species as a whole.

Gender differentiation was believed to have the opposite effect on male evolution. As men became more "masculine" they became ever more detached from their own sexuality and were increasingly able to concentrate on abstract thought. Freed from the tyranny of their "lower instincts" men were said to be able to give themselves over to the high-minded affairs of intellectual, political and economic life. Thus the white male's progressive evolution carried along the entire race while necessarily situating women and non-whites in stagnant or regressive roles.

The even more misogynist view of this theory equated biological reproduction with the degenerating effects of feminine desire and sexuality upon the male and thereby the species. This made the female a symbol of the flesh and species degeneration, and therefore an unsuitable image, muse or vehicle for the ideal. Taken to the extreme, it meant the dangers posed by women to the health of the male body and spirit had to be completely avoided. As a result, nineteenth-century artists and thinkers elevated the image of adolescent girls, and particularly boys, as ideal symbols free from enervating feminine sexuality. As Bram Dijkstra states:

> A new admiration developed for the special beauty of the male. Man, it was now argued, with numerous quotations from Plato, had all the "soft," physical attractions of woman, plus the male's exclusive capacity for intellectual transcendence. The ephebe, the sensitive male adolescent, not woman, was the true ideal of aesthetic beauty. (199)

This shift away from women was further facilitated by the philosophical and evolutionary notion, later championed by Otto Weininger in *Sex and Character*, that, as the male genius continued to distinguish itself from the feminine and grew, it encompassed the totality of human experience, including the masculine and the feminine. The universally evolved white-male was deemed to be a microcosm of human experience who could stand alone as a "monad" of vital integrity.

This characteristically turn-of-the-century vision of evolutionary male transcendence is decidedly present in *Ariel*. In fact, the opening of Prospero's lecture begins with a reference to the physical, bodily manifestation of his speech, the statue of Ariel which he invokes as his "numen." Even before Prospero speaks, this icon of male youth is described as if its physical properties contain the message soon to be transmitted by the professor's lecture:

> Desplegadas las alas; suelta y flotante la leve vestidura, que la
> caricia de la luz en el bronce damasquinaba de oro; erguida la
> amplia frente; entreabiertos los labios por serena sonrisa, todo
> en la actitud de Ariel acusaba admirablemente el gracioso
> arranque del vuelo; y con inspiración dichosa, el arte que había
> dado firmeza escultural a su imagen, había acertado a conservar
> en ella, al mismo tiempo, la apariencia seráfica y la levedad
> ideal. (1)

This is a curious description which underscores the lithe, di-
aphanous qualities of a seemingly non-corporal body. However, this
emphasis on the light, floating and seraphic properties of this body
are offset by other anatomical allusions to an "amplia frente"
(which Prospero "acarició") and an open smiling mouth, which
give the image a tactile bodily presence. Of course this is not the
description of a *living* body but rather of an inanimate sculpture. In
fact, throughout the text there are no direct references to an actual
body that has not been mediated through some literary or sculptural referent. Even when Rodó attempts to conjure up a pseudo-
historical image of classical youth as the archetype of humanist integration of body and mind he cannot help but ground this allusion
in the idea of sculpture:

> Atenas supo engrandecer a la vez el sentido de lo ideal, la razón
> y el instinto, las fuerzas del espíritu y las del cuerpo. Cinceló las
> cuatro fases del alma. Cada ateniense libre describe en derredor
> de sí, para contener su acción, un círculo perfecto, en el que
> ningún desordenado impulso quebrantará la graciosa proporción
> de la línea. Es atleta y escultura viviente en el gimnasio, ciu-
> dadano en el Pnix, polemista y pensador en los pórticos. (11)

Rodó's imaginary Athenian youth is able to control any disorderly
passion which threatens to undermine the threshold of his sexual
self-control because he is indeed a living sculpture, an inanimate yet
living being. This mediation displaces Rodó's anxiety concerning
the body and the Platonic pedagogical relationship to a "safer," de-
eroticized and acceptable level.

Yet the function of the statue of Ariel in the text, which as the
narrator states "dominaba en la sala," cannot be solely attributed to
the peculiar eccentricities, anxiety and repression of a single author
such as Rodó. On the contrary, the ambivalent character of youthful

male statuary has been an extremely productive vehicle for the formation and articulation of a visual and discursive construction of modern nationalism for centuries. One of the foundational texts of this politicized inflection of the aesthetic was itself a work of Classical art history, J.J. Winckelmann's *History of Ancient Art* (1774). In this text Winckelmann linked the linear and smooth lines of youthful Hellenic statuary to the virility of the youthful nation (Mosse 15). Adding to this tradition of German interest in Hellenic statues, Nietzsche also linked classical sculpture of the male body with chaste beauty nearly a hundred years later in *The Case of Wagner* (1871). His split of the Hellenic spirit into a restrained, sculptural Apollinian aspect and its sensual, musical Dionysian opposite underscored the association of male statues with disinterested beauty and masculine discipline. Winckelmann and Nietzsche, as would Rodó, expressed the ideal of self-development and self-control through the image of adolescent male statuary. Accordingly, the sensuality inherent in classical sculpture was replaced with notions of manly self-discipline and healthful abstinence. The sublime was de-eroticized, replacing it with what Rodó calls in *Ariel* "la casta desnudez de las estatuas" (19).

Not only was adolescent male statuary associated with the nation, it was also linked to the notion of national health. The vigorous, lithe, sun and air-soaked bodies of Greek statuary were used as the basis for the emerging ideal national stereotypes. Notions of aesthetic beauty derived from re-written Classical standards influenced the growing sciences of physiognomy, evolution and anthropology which empirically evaluated the "health" of specific "races" according to aesthetic anatomical proportions (Mosse 31). The purportedly "sexless" beauty of Caucasian youth was the measure of health and in itself a healing agent and principle of national organization. Opposite this ideal stood the perceived threats of anatomically different women and allegedly malformed and degenerate ethnic groups or nations.

In *Ariel* we observe the juxtaposition of these two images of health and illness. The statue of Ariel is described as a classically beautiful, linear sculpture bathed in a healing ray of light. Once again the connection to Nietzsche's vision of Apollo, whom he called "the sculptor god," comes to mind. Nietzsche refers to Apollo as the "shining one," and as "the deity of light" whose eye is "sunlike" (*The Case* 35). In keeping with our consideration of

Rodó's description of the statue of Ariel, the sun-drenched quality of Nietzsche's Apollo is also ascribed healing qualities.

The rejuvenating properties of light at work in *Ariel* are also analogous to the medical connotations surrounding ventilation and the aerist thought affiliated with the namesake and figure of Ariel. Nineteenth-century medical science paid increasing attention to the beneficial properties of natural light. As Corbin states, this attention was as morally oriented as it was medically driven:

> But there was increased concern for light in private dwellings, as in public space; this was the beginning of the great swing in attitudes that was to give uncontested supremacy to the visual. Moreover, Baudelocque noted that dark places made flesh soft, puffy and flaccid; inadequate light slowed circulation, brought on the young girl's terrible chlorosis; Jean Starobinski has stressed its effect on the imagination. Darkness made nocturnal animals sad and perfidious; uncertain light was a threat to health, zeal for work, and sexual morality. (154)

In the few textual references to the statue of Ariel Rodó situates the figure in relation to light: "la caricia de la luz en el bronce damasquinaba de oro..."; "bien la esclarecedora penetración del rayo de luz..."; youthful energy and spirit is associated with "movimiento y la luz," and the closing of the essay corresponds to the end of day and the waning of light: "Un rayo del moribundo sol atravesaba la estancia, en medio de discreta penumbra, y tocando la frente de bronce de la estatua, parecía animar en los altivos ojos de Ariel la chispa inquieta de la vida" (59).

Near the end of *Ariel* Rodó does manage to approximate an invocation of an organic, living body without references to inanimate statuary. It happens in Prospero's cautionary remarks to his students regarding the degenerative threats facing Latin America's great cities, which he had already inscribed into the organicist model by referring to them as an "organismo." The debilitating forces which threaten to weaken these cities are those of technological modernization and massification. Yet paradoxically, the feared end-result of these enervating modern forces is not compared to a modern European city but to the traditional Western paradigm of decadence, the Oriental city-states of Sidon, Tyre and Carthage. Against this contagion Rodó invokes the collective physiognomical body of his students as an antidote: "A vuestra generación toca impedirlo; a la juventud que se levanta, sangre y músculo y nervio del porvenir. Quiero considerarla personificada en vosotros" (53). Here Rodó's vision of youth is not an abstract exhortation about self-conscious faith, but a direct reference to the temporal and anatomical condition of his students. Nevertheless, like his references to male statuary, this bodily citation refers to a non-existent, fictional body, for it is addressed to an imaginary audience and not to a live constituency. Prospero concludes his lecture by connecting these fictional referents of youth through the statue of Ariel. In this way Rodó also provides structural closure to his essay by ending Prospero's lecture with a declaration that subjugates its rhetorical content to the visual image of Ariel's youth: "Aún más que mi palabra, yo exijo de vosotros un dulce e indeleble recuerdo para mi estatua de Ariel. Yo quiero que la imagen leve y graciosa de este bronce se imprima desde ahora en la más segura intimidad de vuestro espíritu" (58).

MASCULINE REGENERATION AND THE EVOLUTIONARY FANTASY OF *ARIEL*

It is somehow fitting that Rodó's references to the therapeutic qualities of the adolescent male's body, spirit and internal life force are based upon imaginary, inanimate and literary images of youth. The statues, literary protagonists and fictional students of the text are as intangible and non-existent as the figure and therapeutic program embodied by Ariel. Ariel, as a Latin American subject, as an allegory for national regeneration, does not exist. Ariel, the symbol of health and rejuvenation, is a hypothesized, precarious evolutionary outcome contingent upon the healthy or sickly beliefs and practices of Latin American youth.

Rodó's anxiety concerning the possibilities for Latin American regeneration reflects his ambivalent feelings about the evolutionary model. A conceptual linkage between the brutally accelerating differentiation of the species, divisive social heterogeneity and excessive division of labor threatens to fragment or restrict the integral personality of the youthful individual and society:

> Quiere, en efecto, la ley de la evolución, manifestándose en la sociedad como en la naturaleza por una creciente tendencia a la

heterogeneidad, que, a medida que la cultura general de las sociedades avanza, se limite correlativamente la extensión de las
aptitudes individuales y haya de ceñirse el campo de acción de
cada uno a una especialidad más restringida. (10)

Rodó's concern with the brutality of the evolutionary process
can be traced back to the predatory evolutionary models established by Darwin and Spencer. Phrases such as "the survival of the
fittest" paraphrased a theory which pitted the individual progress
of superior species or races against a greater collective decline of inferior groups. Therefore, evolutionary progress necessarily indicated greater degrees of social and economic inequality within society. In fact, conflict itself, whether it be between the "sexes," ethnic
groups or social classes, gave evidence of a vitally operative evolutionary system. In *Ariel* this positive appraisal of conflict is given its
philosophical equivalent in the Hegelian thesis-antithesis model of
history: "...las grandes evoluciones de la historia, las grandes
épocas, los períodos más luminosos y fecundos en el desenvolvimiento de la humanidad, son casi siempre la resultante de dos
fuerzas distintas co-actuales, que mantienen, por los concertados
impulsos de su oposición, el interés y el estímulo de la vida..." (37).

The precondition for this combative progress is an ever intensi-
fying internal heterogeneity or differentiation within the species.
Such a process inescapably involves questions of quantity and quality in a mutually antagonistic and dependent relationship. The natural selection of the few requires the distinction from the many.
Thus paradoxically, the healthy advance of the race was declared to
be dependent on the degeneration of the majority, a potentially
dangerous condition to be overcome, for the benefit of the entire
species, by the superior minority. Just how to ensure the health and
predominance of this select minority is the central concern of Rodó
in *Ariel*:

> Si la aparición y el florecimiento, en la sociedad, de las más ele-
> vadas actividades humanas, de las que determinan la alta cultura,
> requieren como condición indispensable la existencia de una
> población cuantiosa y densa, es precisamente porque esa impor-
> tancia cuantitativa de la población, dando lugar a la más comple-
> ja división del trabajo, posibilita la formación de fuertes elemen-
> tos dirigentes que hagan efectivo el dominio de la *calidad* sobre
> el *número*. (26)

In the larger context of the aesthetically coded yet organicist terminology of *Ariel*, this passage about democracy indicates that the regenerative, evolutionary figure of Ariel cannot exist without the degenerate threat of Caliban.

Aside from its obvious connection to degeneracy and evolutionary theory, another striking feature of this formula of a qualitatively
select minority overcoming and benefitting a necessarily impover-
ished and biologically inferior majority is its convergence with liberal, market oriented economic theory. In this sense the evolutionary
"struggle for existence" is analogous to the "free" competition of
the market. In this light it is helpful to recall the historical foundation of evolutionary theory in the pessimistic economic and demog-
raphic studies of Robert Malthus (Stuart C. Gilman 176).

In *Ariel*, Rodó hopes that a carefully guided democracy, one
which will not degenerate "en nivelador igualitarismo," (32) will at-
tenuate the harshness of evolutionary and social competition. Just
as the market is said to select and enrich those whose innate talents
and intelligence are best suited to it, Rodó asserts that the social
conditions of political democracy enable the naturally meritorious
to rise above the majority. Therefore, despite his distrust of democracy Rodó proposes it as the system which will most efficiently and
scientifically select the naturally superior:

> Racionalmente concebida, la democracia admite siempre un im-
> prescriptible elemento aristocrático, que consiste en establecer la
> superioridad de los mejores, ... Ella consagra como las aristocra-
> cias, la distinción de calidad; pero las resuelve a favor de las cali-
> dades realmentes superiores, –las de la virtud, el carácter, el es-
> píritu.... (32)

Nevertheless, the dangers of social leveling and species degeneration inherent in democracy hang over Latin America. Following
Fouillée, Rodó asserts that as biological and social systems pro-
gressed, the brutal competition of natural selection would diminish
(Brotherston 6). This hopeful evolutionary result is contingent
upon the moral and healthy comportment of youth. If Latin America's youth believes in itself, shuns the illness of "nordomanía," re-
stricts itself to the chaste, exclusively male contemplation of the
ideal, itself the tautological construct of male beauty, then the conserved, fecund and sexually charged vital internal force of youth

will act as a catalyst and accelerate the pace of evolution. If Prospero's students are patient and avoid immediate "consagración" or gratification, their "energía viril tendrá con ello un estímulo más poderoso..." (55), permitting them "...trabajar en beneficio del porvenir, para que acelerada la evolución por el esfuerzo de los hombres, llegue con ella con más rápido impulso a su término final..." (57). This declaration that human behavior can intervene in the process of biological and social evolution once again situates Rodó within one of the basic premises of degeneracy theory, namely, the Lamarckian theory of evolutionary change based on the transmission of negative or positive acquired traits to subsequent generations.

Rodó actually describes the male youth's contribution of its vital life-force to the species as an evolutionary act. Youth will serve as an intermediate species between stages of development, what he calls a "premature" and "prophetic species." The regenerative qualities of youth are further described in the terminology used to analyze the emergence of a new species from a randomly isolated and successful mutation or variety to an established and dominant species: "El tipo nuevo empieza por significar, apenas diferencias individuales y aisladas; los individualismos se organizan más tarde en 'variedad'; y, por último, la variedad encuentra para propagarse un medio que la favorece, y entonces ella asciende quizá al rango específico..." (55). After becoming firmly established in a new evolutionary stage, the prophetic species of youth will extend itself and govern: "el grupo se hace muchedumbre y reina."

Despite the assertion that the figure of Ariel is an imagined, evolutionary possibility, Rodó makes the biological inevitability of this possibility visible in the language of the text. That is to say, despite the aesthetic and rhetorically stylized character of Rodó's discourse, it nevertheless links the aesthetic to an organicist model through images which situate idealist or spiritual transcendence within a larger framework of species evolution. This textual performance of the evolutionary paradigm is achieved, paradoxically, in the terminology which is supposedly the most vehement in its rejection of the body. I am referring specifically to the language pertaining to the binary opposition between the "high" and the "low."

As I have argued earlier, this spatial metaphor is grounded in a division of the body into the regenerative, caucasian, masculine, and "high" organ of the brain, personified by Ariel, and the degenerate, non-white and feminine "low" of the sexual and excremental organs embodied by Caliban. In terms of language, the evolutionary transition from Caliban to Ariel is constructed as a process of ascension wherein the species achieves increasingly greater states of control over its body, thereby reaching a higher state of evolutionary development. Rodó creates this effect through the constant use of verbs, nouns and adjectives which indicate upward movement away from the earth and the body (Caliban) and into the sky.

The initial presentation of Caliban and Ariel posits them within this process of species elevation. Ariel, whose wings literally allow him to fly upwards towards evolutionary perfection triumphs over the "bajos estímulos" of Caliban to become "el término ideal a que asciende la selección humana..." The cluster "término ideal" situates ideal or aesthetic perfection within a process of species evolution which produces Ariel as its highest form, its biological and aesthetic limit. This is the goal towards which natural selection, "la selección humana" is rising, "asciende."

Natural and spiritual selection are equated with the "enaltecimiento de la vida" which is generated by scientifically aloof "estímulos desinteresados" (25). After citing Spencer, Rodó depicts a socially evolved nation in lofty visual, topographical and literary terms which connect the ascension of the Darwinian ladder of species advancement with mental or phrenological development of the brain: "los pueblos que han alcanzado un perfecto desenvolvimiento de su genio presiden al glorioso coronamiento de su obra,... terminando en olímpico sosiego, la ascensión poderosa, más arriba de las cumbres de la Cordillera" (51). In this passage all terms point either to the top of the body, "genio," "coronamiento" and its craniological development, "desenvolvimiento;" or to the process of evolutionary ascension or completion: "terminando," "coronamiento," "terminando," "olímpico," "ascención," and "cumbres." From its "alteza divina" the "vestments" of a spiritually evolved nation can "elevar a quien las posee por encima de las cosas vulgares" (51), and the evolved "flota por encima de la muchedumbre" (52). Prospero's exhortation to his students that they believe in America's regeneration is enunciated in an image that situates the rejuvenation of the region as an evolutionary goal hovering over the present like a stained glass window above a church interior: "Pensad en ella a lo menos; el honor de vuestra historia futura depende que tengáis constantemente ante los ojos del alma la visión de esa

América regenerada, cerniéndose a lo alto sobre las realidades del presente, como en la nave gótica el vasto rosetón que arde en luz sobre lo austero de los muros sombríos" (54). This inspired youth, following the biological model of Dr. Oswald Heer,[30] will "ascend" to a new evolutionary level, or "rango específico," to establish a higher plane of being (55).

This mixing of aesthetic idealism and evolutionary science was a particularly productive discursive modality of the turn-of-the-century. Rodó's formulation of a spiritual-evolutionary regeneration and transcendence in *Ariel* is comparable to the North American natural scientist Joseph Le Conte's (1823-1901) synthesis of Neo-platonic idealism and evolutionary science. Le Conte, in his book *Evolution: Its Nature, Its Evidences, and Its Relation to Religious Thought* (1888-91), postulated a transformation of materiality into life-force which would enable humanity to break with its bodily and material limitations in order to reach a higher plane of mind. The intersection between a natural scientist like Le Conte and a man-of-letters like Rodó is striking if we consider Bram Dijkstra's analysis of Le Conte's theory: "Ultimately the transcendence of man into the realm of the ideal would be his liberation from, would constitute his being 'lifted above,' the world of the 'earth-mother' into the higher plane of the masculine spirit" (Dijkstra 217). This description accurately describes the theory of spatially ascending, male, evolutionary transcendence and degeneration which I have been investigating in *Ariel*. In Rodó's terms, the future health of Latin America depends on the outcome of a struggle between Caliban, who represents the degenerative constituencies of the earth-mother, and Ariel, who personifies the rejuvenating qualities of the masculine intellect.

Near the end of Prospero's lecture Rodó synthesizes the evolutionary and Neo-platonic idealism invested in the figure of Ariel. It is a *crescendo* which defines Ariel both in terms of what he signifies in terms of nature, that is, his rank in the evolution of the species, and in terms of his spiritual meaning. Rodó grounds this culmination of the organicist and aesthetic intersection of the text through the use of a language of rising teleological inevitability: "Ariel es,

---

[30] According to Brotherston, Rodó's conception of youth as a prophetic species was in part derived from Heer's work mediated through his reading of Quinet's translation. See Brotherston, n. 1, p. 97.

para la Naturaleza, el excelso coronamiento de su obra, que hace terminarse el proceso de ascensión de las formas organizadas, con la llamarada del espíritu" (57). Ariel is hypothesized as the highest evolutionary form in nature, the ascending, crowning glory of its competitive process of species ("las formas organizadas") differentiation, advancement and/or reversion. Ariel's role as an evolutionary vanguard is given a historically resonant if not mythological literary agency; Rodó calls him "el héroe epónimo en la epopeya de la especie" who has inspired the "primer hombre prehistórico" and the "ayra primitivo" until he evolved into the biologically inflected "razas superiores" (57). The motivating force behind Ariel's therapeutic ascension, "el movimiento ascendente de la vida," is the properly invested and controlled life-force of adolescent youth. As Rodó establishes in the initial classroom setting of the text, the proper investment of this life-force is the contemplation of the ideal in the chaste company of fellow male students and a male teacher-mentor. In this way Rodó links his proposal for pan-American regeneration to a sensually charged yet rigidly chaste masculine enclave of learning and introspection. As an antidote to European decadence, on the one hand, and as a remedy for North American utilitarianism on the other, *Ariel* became a fundamental guide to Latin American intellectuals seeking to define and defend a Latin American cultural identity. Yet the therapeutic program proposed in *Ariel* is plagued by anxiety concerning the potential for excessive self-absorption and homosexuality within Rodó's idealized and repressed vision of male bonding. It is this recurrent anxiety which reveals Rodó's uncertainty about the health of his own program for Latin American regeneration.

ALCIDES ARGUEDAS' *PUEBLO ENFERMO*:
THE TERMINALLY ILL NATION

THE NATIONAL, PAN-AMERICAN AND SPANISH ROOTS
OF *PUEBLO ENFERMO*

In the final section of this investigation of the discourse of national illness in Spain and Latin America, I will discuss *Pueblo enfermo*, Alcides Arguedas' essay on Bolivia. In many ways it is fitting that I conclude with Arguedas. Firstly, *Pueblo enfermo* (1909) is one of the most clearly stated, unapologetic and condemnatory examples of the essay of national degeneration, therefore, my consideration of it will necessarily reinforce the analysis of Ganivet's and Rodó's relatively conditional (when compared to Arguedas) embrace of this particular kind of analysis. Concepts, examples and narratives of racial and sexual degeneration which are tangentially alluded to or are inscribed within Ganivet's anti-scientific idealism, or obscured by Rodó's spiritual, aestheticized evolutionism, are brought clearly and unhesitatingly into the light of day by Arguedas' uncompromising *Pueblo enfermo*. Like his predecessors, Arguedas will take up the themes of aboulia, the "femininization" of the nation, the sexual draining of male national virility and the comparison of all of the above to the medically condemned, enervating practice of masturbation. Yet unlike Ganivet and Rodó, Arguedas makes this comparison very explicit, thus shedding additional light on his more discreet and supposedly "anti-positivist" or "spiritualist" predecessors.

Arguedas' work shows, moreover, the intimate connection between Spanish and Latin American authors of social organicism and degeneracy theory. Aside from the documentable fact that both of these traditions were substantially influenced by French and English biological and psychological theory, there is also ample evidence, as I noted apropos of Rodó, of direct communication and intellectual sympathy between segments of the finesecular Spanish and Latin American intelligentsia. Arguedas' personal correspondence gives evidence of the close personal and intellectual ties between Spanish authors like Ganivet or Unamuno who proclaimed the "illness" of Spain, and their Latin American counterparts such as Rodó or Arguedas. Specifically, the inspiration, publication and promotion of Arguedas' *Pueblo enfermo* involved the influence and participation of Ramiro de Maeztu, Miguel de Unamuno, Rafael de Altamira and Ricardo Macías Picavea. In his prologue to the 1909 first edition of *Pueblo enfermo* (repeated in later editions as well), Maetzu erroneously claimed credit for himself and his compatriots for initiating the movement of "national" medical introspection and congratulated Arguedas for its continuation in Latin America: "Usted ha hecho por su país, con este libro, lo que unos cuantos españoles hicimos por el nuestro hace diez años, a raíz de haberse perdido las colonias." The fact that Latin American statesmen-authors such as Echeverría, Sarmiento, and Alberdi had already initiated similar discourses in Latin America does not undermine Maeztu's illusion of momentary fraternity.

In a letter written in 1909 shortly after reading a complementary copy of *Pueblo enfermo* sent to him by Arguedas, the Spanish historiographer and author of *Psicología del pueblo español* (1902), Rafael de Altamira, the future writer of the prologue to Arguedas' 1923 edition of his *Raza de Bronce*, waxed enthusiastic about their "común aspiración a penetrar la psicología de las colectividades" (Roca 159). Equally enthusiastic about Arguedas' work was Unamuno, whose psychological approach to national analysis, evident in his *En torno al casticismo* (1895) and other texts, greatly influenced Arguedas and is widely cited throughout *Pueblo enfermo*.

Then there is the case of Ricardo Macías Picavea whose *El problema nacional* (1899) is also cited at length in *Pueblo enfermo* as a literary model for the diagnosis of national illness. Picavea's essay is interesting in that it openly declares the need for medical diagnosis and clinical therapy which writers like Ganivet and Unamuno treat more figuratively, in this sense anticipating Arguedas' own materialism; Picavea declares: "¿Son las angustias de un enfermo las que nos solicitan? Luego a la clínica debemos pedir nuestro pan. Diagnóstico, patogenia, tratamiento: no hay otra manera de proceder" (Ramsden, *1898 Movement* 132).

Nevertheless, the Spanish influence is of ancillary importance in contrast to Arguedas' Bolivian and Latin American precursors and contemporaries in degeneracy theory. In Bolivia, positivism gained importance in the 1870's, becoming the ideology of liberals such as Gabriel René-Moreno and Nicomedes Antelo, the Bolivian promoters of Social Darwinism. These intellectuals viewed the indigenous and hybrid populations of Bolivia as sources of national weakness and as impediments to parliamentary democracy (Fernández 65). They were echoed by Daniel Sánchez Bustamante (1870-1933), an ardent adherent of Spencer who wrote a book on the latter's *Principles of Psychology* in 1903 (Ávila Echazú 90).

Arguedas incorporated the work of these Bolivian thinkers into his own, on occasion citing them by name. In this sense, it is possible to assert that Arguedas' work is a direct continuation of the positivist period in Bolivia, particularly inasmuch as some critics have postulated that Bolivia did not experience a spiritualist, anti-positivist reaction of the sort represented by Rodó or some of the *modernistas* (Francovich 7). Despite this claim there is, as Ávila Echazú notes, evidence of a critical backlash to the unfulfilled promises of positivist thought in Bolivia (89). The position of Arguedas in this debate is somewhat complex. While accepting the bulk of the racial, geographical and evolutionary jargon of the positivists, *Pueblo enfermo* is also an expression of disillusion with the failed pretense of national progress heralded by liberal positivism. In *Pueblo enfermo* there is little hope that improvements in infrastructure and education, components of an overall rationalization of the nation, will bring about the pending stages of evolution proposed by the Comtean model. The hopes for such progress have been dashed by the pessimistic prognosis offered by ethno-psychology and anthropology. Consequently, for Arguedas, the assertion that Bolivia was in the midst of a rationally based period of progress becomes associated with excessive or dishonest political rhetoric and governmental corruption.

Arguedas was not the first Latin American intellectual to lose faith in the promise of scientific, rational progress and evolution in the Americas. Two Argentineans, Agustín Álvarez and Carlos Octavio Bunge, put forth earlier the pessimistic proposal that Latin America's ethnic composition and psychological constitution represented nearly insuperable obstacles to national progress. In his *Manual de patología política* (1899), Álvarez does not posit racial inferiority as the direct consequence of "inferior blood," but rather links national inferiority to deficiencies in ethics, morality and reason. Nevertheless the scientific basis for these shortcomings remains linked to the notion of a racially derived pathology of the will which manifests itself in immoral, irrational and unethical behavior, thus situating Álvarez's ethical critique within the biological racial paradigm.

In Bunge's *Nuestra América* (1903), social organicism, ethnopsychology and geographical determinism are employed to diagnose and cure Argentina's national "illness." For Bunge, the source of Argentina's problems is racial, including its Spanish ancestors as well as its mixed indigenous, mestizo and mulatto populations. Bunge does, however, find hope in the presence of an allegedly superior white minority and the partial evolutionary elimination of the "inferior" mixed and non-white races. This belief is based, in part, on his readings of Lombroso and Nordau who stated that the hybrid races are prone to degenerative alcoholism and infectious disease, pathologies which Bunge praises as nature's way of purging Argentina of allegedly inferior elements.[31] To counter-balance and eventually "absorb" the enervating presence of these allegedly inferior groups, both Bunge and Álvarez encouraged the promotion of European immigration to "whiten" the Americas.

Without a doubt Álvarez and Bunge are the two most important precursors for Arguedas' medical conception of Bolivia's ills, although one could also consider the impact of his friend Manuel Ugarte's *Enfermedades sociales* of 1905. Both Álvarez and Bunge are cited throughout *Pueblo enfermo*, yet it is Bunge's *Nuestra América* which truly seems to have served as a conceptual model. Even at the level of structure and exposition Arguedas' text mimics Bunge's earlier study as Arguedas himself suggests in *Pueblo enfermo*:

> Estos son los principales rasgos de las regiones de Bolivia; pero hay otras comunes a los demás pueblos de la América latina, y cuyo anáysis ha sido perfectamente hecho por Octavio Bunge en

---

[31] Celebrating the mortality inflicted by these illnesses and vices Bunge states: "Además, el alcoholismo, la viruela y la tubercolosis, –¡benditos sean!– habían diezmado a la población indígena y africana de la provincia-capital, depurando sus elementos étnicos, europeizándolos, españolizándolos."

su excelente obra *Nuestra América*, y a la que es preciso recurrir si se quieren conocer y comprender las variaciones de ese carácter tornadizo y de manifestaciones incoherentes. (87)

In addition to this matrix of Spanish and Latin American influences, it is necessary to consider the direct impact of French, English and German degeneracy theory upon Arguedas' thought. The list of European historiographers, philosophers, psychologists and novelists cited by Arguedas in *Pueblo enfermo* is quite long and repeats many of the figures of nineteenth-century thought reviewed in my previous discussions of Ganivet and Rodó. Nevertheless, we also discover other sources decidedly absent in Ganivet and Rodó. Among the authors liberally cited in *Pueblo enfermo* are the following famous, and in some cases, infamous names: Bagehot, Bourget, Carlyle, Flaubert, Fouillée, Guyau, Hitler (in the 1937 edition), Le Bon, Lombroso, Macaulay, Nietzsche, Nordau, Ruskin, Schopenhauer, Taine and Zola. When asked to characterize his reading preferences Arguedas replied: "Soy como la abeja que coge miel de todas las flores" (Albarracín Millán 140). From this mixed bag of sources Arguedas developed his own theoretical blend of geographical determinism, racial psychology and pathology, misogyny, scientific anti-democratic thought and sexual degeneration theory. Moreover, Arguedas' readings and admiration for certain authors also affected his personal sense of self and his relationship to his own work and society. This was especially true in the case of the German philosophers Nietzsche and Schopenhauer. From both of these philosophers Arguedas found support for his own pessimism and misanthropy. In Schopenhauer Arguedas found a model for relentless self-critique and introspection, while in Nietzsche Arguedas discovered the kindred spirit of the critic who bursts others' idealist illusions, thus fashioning for himself the role of national provocateur.

Arguedas reproduced the multifaceted and multi-disciplinary nature of his diverse intellectual formation in his own work. He wrote and received both acclaim and criticism as a novelist, journalist, sociologist and historian. Moreover, in a manner that has been indicative of the relationship of scholarship to politics in Latin America throughout its history, Arguedas compounded his intellectual interests by holding governmental positions as a diplomat and as a politician. In this way Arguedas is a prime example of the nine-

teenth century Latin American man-of-letters who operated in a social, cultural and political atmosphere characterized by the integration of cultural and political discourses and the absence of a decisive split between the cultural and political intelligentsia.

Indeed, *Pueblo enfermo* itself, which can be narrowly defined as
a sociological text, is in reality methodologically and generically a
heterogeneous text containing an eclectic range of discourses reflecting the diversity of Arguedas' erudition and personal experiences. *Pueblo enfermo* includes instances of literary *costumbrismo*,
literary criticism, psychology, sexology, biology, geography, political
science and historiography.[32]

Arguedas brings the heterogeneous nature of the essay as a
form, together with his multiple discursive methodologies and personal experience, to *Pueblo enfermo*. Nevertheless, there are obvious ideological problems and methodological shortcomings in the
text. The racial concepts and simplistic psychological theories employed in the text are as outdated as they are despicable. Yet other
discourses, such as that of the public health reformer who seeks to
improve the nutrition of his people, reduce their substance abuse
and raise their hygienic standards, remain very much a part of our
present political rhetoric both to the right and the left of the political spectrum.

This ambivalence between racism and reformism is further
complicated by the historical circumstances surrounding the publication of *Pueblo enfermo*. In the decades prior to the publication
Pueblo enfermo, Bolivia had been devastated by a series of ethnic
and civil wars culminating in 1899 Revolution. The destruction and
hatreds engendered by these conflicts were still very much in effect
when the text appeared. One of the main and unresolved causes of
the conflicts, was the ruthless exploitation and degradation of the
indigenous population under a system of virtual slavery. The harshness of the Indian's living conditions, the paucity of its nutrition,

---

[32] Ultimately, this discursively heterogeneous character of *Pueblo enfermo* can
be linked to the nature of the essay as a genre in a more general sense. It is the
openness of the genre which facilitates the mixture of subjective ideologies, aesthetic style and supposedly objective forms of knowledge. This mixture is characterized
by the explicit presence of the author in the text in the role of intellectual and existential authority. This authority is a function of the essayist's appropriation of the
discourses of the natural and social sciences which he/she combines to form a discursively complex genre of exposition or persuasion.

and the poor state of their health was documented by Arguedas in *Pueblo enfermo*, along with the government's official indifference to, and corrupt profit from, their plight.

The decline in the living conditions of the indigenous communities of Bolivia at the end of the nineteenth century was directly linked to the ongoing assault on the traditional colonial system of Indian tribute based on collective landholdings and contributions. As early as 1825, liberal reformers sought to "individualize" the Indian contribution to the national coffers by imposing a direct tax on the sources and tools of production and exchange (Platt 285). Throughout the century, the Indians' productive and political autonomy was threatened by the privatization of communal lands, taxation and the penetration of mestizo peasants on their *ayllus*. The indigenous resistance to these encroachments on their traditional status and relative autonomy led to violent confrontations between increasingly coordinated indigenous communities and liberal regimes intent on imposing their vision of national progress.

In this sense there was a real social, racial, economic, cultural and political crisis in Bolivia at the beginning of the twentieth century when Arguedas wrote *Pueblo enfermo*. That many of the problems described by Arguedas were real is not in doubt nor the issue of this investigation. What will be of concern is the way in which Arguedas perceived this reality. Arguedas did not ascribe this crisis to larger social and economic forces at work in the nation, such as the penetration of foreign capital and political leverage at the end of the nineteenth century or the social displacements, migrations and adjustments initiated by the forced transition to a relatively liberalized, modern and dependent economy. Rather, Arguedas viewed the crisis facing Bolivia as the inevitable result of its long-standing biological and racial character. It is this medicalization of underdevelopment, and not the reality of underdevelopment itself, that I will challenge in this account of *Pueblo enfermo*.

RACIAL PSYCHOLOGY AND ILLNESS

For Arguedas, the history of a nation is indistinguishable from that of the individuals who compose it. Importantly, Arguedas does not examine individual and national psychologies as reactive manifestations to socio-economic history, nor does he consider them as co-functional catalysts for historical stagnation or transformation, rather, he views them as the absolute causative force behind all historical conflicts, exchanges and processes.

The premise for this belief is that individual and group morality is the psychological component which guides historical development. Depending on the nature of this morality, its deployment can result in either the improvement or detriment of the nation. It is the character of this morality, its vitality or sluggishness, which allows or inhibits the development of reason, the conceptual foundation of enlightenment and the precondition for progress and modernization.

For Arguedas, morality is inescapably tied to heredity and race. Here he was following the school of thought known as anthroposociology, which associated the social and cultural progress or regression of peoples to their race (Stabb 13). The key figure of this school for Arguedas, whom he cites in *Pueblo enfermo*, was Gustave Le Bon. In his *The Psychology of Peoples* (1894), Le Bon declared that each race possesses its own distinct psychology. Furthermore, Le Bon established a racial hierarchy which classified the races in terms of physiognomy, intellect and morality. For both Le Bon and Arguedas the European was the superior race against which all other "races" were measured (Stabb 13).

Of course as a Latin American, and specifically as a Bolivian, Arguedas did not need to wait for a turn-of-the-century French ethno-psychologist and social organicist to establish a racial social pyramid for the population of Latin America. In fact, the hierarchical division of race in Arguedas' *Pueblo enfermo* does not differ substantially from the social and racial paradigm introduced into Latin America by Spanish colonialism, illustrating a continuity characterized by Albarracín Millán as "una aceptación llana del cuadro colonial que introdujo el racismo español: la superioridad de la raza blanca, el proceso inferior de la mestización y la inferioridad indígena" (146). In this sense, the modern raciologist's criteria for classifications of difference and quality represent a biological, discursive modernization of colonial Spain's aristocratic proto-scientific obsession with the racial, expressed in the doctrine of "limpieza de sangre."

At the beginning of the chapter titled "Psicología de la raza indígena," Arguedas introduces what appears to be a contradiction into his race-based psychology. He seems to challenge the biological category of race itself:

> El término *raza*, usado así de modo tan categórico para determinar la ligera variación que existe entre los grupos pobladores del suelo boliviano, parece fuera de lugar, y mucho más si se tienen en cuenta las restricciones y reservas que hoy día suscita su uso por no conceptuársele categóricamente valorizado por la ciencia ni creer que determine de manera concreta sus alcances, pues, según Novicow, 'nadie ha podido decir jamás cuáles rasgos establecían las características de la raza'. (31)

Arguedas compounds this theoretical challenge to the notion of race with observations on the social reality of racial mixing in Bolivia, a process that has blurred the lines between the races. Thus, Arguedas states, the issue of racial assignation in Bolivia is based on social convention or *class* (a term Arguedas would not employ), a distinction linked to what he calls the "figuración social." In light of these historical and theoretical obstacles, Arguedas declares that his consideration of race will be limited to a psychological point of view: "Es, pues, entonces a este solo precio, es decir, al de considerar las *razas* sólo desde el punto de vista *psicológico* y para mayor facilidad expositiva que, con pequeña variación, acepto la clasificación establecida por los autores del censo" (33).

Arguedas' apparent problematization of the category of race and its conflation with the more acceptable discipline of psychology can only be viewed as an example of defensive double speak. The kind of ethnic psychology or anthroposociology practiced by Arguedas was premised upon a biological model of race. What Arguedas alleges to be the "psychological" traits of the different races are directly explained through references to biological processes of racial degeneration. Moreover, as Martin Stabb reminds us, by the time of the definitive 1937 edition of *Pueblo enfermo*, Arguedas' raciological theories had become so entrenched in his thought that he went so far as to include citations from the Spanish translation of Hitler's *Mein Kampf*.

For Arguedas, the paradox of abundant natural resources and national underdevelopment could only be explained by the racial and psychological inferiority of Bolivia's population. The main source of this inferiority, Arguedas maintains, and the primary obstacle to progress in Bolivia is, and has always been, the indigenous population:

De no haber predominio de sangre indígena, desde el comienzo habría dado el país orientación consciente a su vida, adoptando toda clase de perfeciones en el orden material y moral y, estaría hoy en el mismo nivel que muchos pueblos más favorecidos por corrientes inmigratorios venidas del viejo continente. (32)

Arguedas' explanation of the Indian population's inferiority involves a contradictory mixture of grudging admiration and outright contempt. This ambivalence in Arguedas' attitude towards the Indians can be traced to the mixed modalities of degenerative thought he uses to explain their debased state. Some of the arguments which Arguedas employs link their deficiencies to historical psychological and physiological degradations they suffered beginning with the conquest and continuing through the development of *latifundismo* and mining up to Arguedas' lifetime. This discourse of exploitative mistreatment and acquired degenerative traits does, at times, engender a sympathetic, reformist tone in Arguedas' analysis. Other alleged psychological features of the Indian psychology, however, those which Arguedas characterizes as non-historical, innate and incurable, lead to a condemning discourse of congenital corruption.

This contradictory vision of the Indian population is situated within a larger matrix of conceptual equations and oppositions. Arguedas makes an analogy between the indigenous population and nature, at the same time establishing a rupture between Indian culture and (European) civilization. In terms of Bolivian geography, this semantic series locates viable, legitimate indigenous culture in the countryside while simultaneously denouncing urban indigenous inhabitants as a degenerate impediment to progress.[33] This socially, economically and culturally motivated geographical separation of the races in Bolivia was also sanctioned by degeneracy theory. As Nancy Stepan has stated, nineteenth-century racial biologists linked the health of a race to its geographical point of origin (98-99). To break with these origins was to invite degeneration. This led to the assertion that non-white peoples were by their "nature" non-cosmopolitan. Thus, for Arguedas, the presence of Indians in Bolivia's cities portended their biological and cultural decomposition.

---

[33] Albarracín Millán has described this attitude in the following way: "Por una parte una abierta hostilidad ante la presencia de los indios en las ciudades y por otra una franca simpatía por el indio agricultor que trabaja en el campo" (91).

The underlying theme of this contradictory vision is Arguedas' notion concerning the loss of cultural "purity" or "innocence," or what in anthropological terms would be called acculturation. Arguedas' notion of purity is tied into a geographic relationship between the indigenous "race" and its natural environment. As a member of the urban, land-owning elite Arguedas admires the indigenous population when it is limited to what he considers to be its proper place, the countryside. His descriptions of the rural Indian speak of the latter's abuse under the system of *latifundista* servitude or "pongueaje." They reflect an attitude of grudging admiration for the silent suffering and physical and mental toughness of indigenous men and women under harsh, unjust conditions. But such sympathetic moments are often grounded in terms which undermine Arguedas' construction of a noble and stoic indigenous martyrdom by comparing the Indians' endurance to the mute, hardened insensitivity of animals, as in the image of their calloused feet, which he describes as "dura como casco de caballo." Again comparing the Indian to an animal, Arguedas argues that the Indian can only socialize with his own kind or species: "es animal expansivo con los de su especie; fuera de su centro, mantiénese reservado y hosco" (36). In his use of the term "species" Arguedas reproduces one of Social Darwinism's basic conceptual confusions, the interchangeability of the terms "race" and "species" within the competitive evolutionary struggle. As Raymond Williams has argued, this confusion of terminology is central to scientifically "justified" imperialist ideology, where Darwin's doctrine of the "survival of the fittest" explains colonial conquest and subjugation as natural, biological processes of competition. Furthermore, as Williams points out, according to this ideology the stronger race (read: imperialist power) has a moral obligation to fulfill its biological destiny and to ignore artificial ethical or legal restraints (92-93).

According to Arguedas, a principal sign of the indigenous population's evolutionary primitiveness was its supposed lack of sexual differentiation in the division of labor and social responsibility. After listing the physical hardships suffered by the Indian male Arguedas says that: "La mujer observa la misma vida y, en ocasiones, sus faenas son más rudas." As a result of this social integration, the indigenous woman does not conceive of herself in the purely domestic and aesthetic terms of a Western or Westernized bourgeoisie. As Arguedas states: "ni concibe ni gusta de las exquisiteces propias del sexo." Although Arguedas views this unevolved, gender-inclusive, non-division of labor as a sign of cultural, social and biological backwardness, he nevertheless finds it to be perfectly suitable to the Indian "species," just as he deems the typically "non-feminine" traits, aggressiveness, strength and bravery, to be natural for Indian women but not for women of other racial or social groups. In fact, Arguedas respects this female strength and purity of the Indian woman and compares her favorably with middle class and oligarchical women: "Desconoce esas enfermedades de que están llenas nuestras mujeres por el abuso del corsé y el demasiado gasto de perfumes y polvos. Sus nervios no vibran con el dolor ni el placer" (39). In other words, Arguedas infers, the Indian woman might be inferior but at least she is not hysterical.

In *Pueblo enfermo* the unevolved, animal primitiveness of Indian psychology is given a basis in geographical determinism. For Arguedas there is little distinction between nature and the Indian: "La pampa y el indio no forman sino una sola entidad" (34). The collective psychology of a regional tribe is determined by its immediate topographical environment. The harsh weather and physical monotony of the *altiplano* allegedly give the Indian a severe, unemotional, non-aesthetic, pessimistic and abulic personality in a manner reminiscent of Naturalism and its sense of the relation between environment and personality.

For Arguedas the harshness of the physical environment is mimicked by indigenous culture under the conditions imposed by feudal servitude. In Arguedas' account, Indian children are born into a cold, unhygienic environment where they are put in with the livestock. Here among the animals the child is introduced to the Darwinian struggle among the species in a fight for their shared food. Finally leaving this space of shared human and animal excrement, the child takes on even tougher responsibilities.

According to Arguedas, this supposedly harsh upbringing instills a profound sense of sadness in the indigenous population which can manifest itself in passivity, or, in what is worse for the country, in the Nietzschean resentment of the downtrodden: "Y comienzan a ser hombres, a saber que la vida es triste y a sentir germinar dentro de sí el odio contra los blancos, ese odio inextinguible y consciente porque nace de la crueldad que éstos usan con los suyos" (37). With this kind of psychological argument Arguedas seeks to explain the protracted civil and racial wars which racked Bolivia in the mid and late nineteenth century.

Through the combination of a cruel physical environment, an equally severe upbringing, the allegedly corrupting influence of Indian priests or *yatiris* and the abuse of landowners and government officials, Arguedas states that the Indian spirit becomes corrupted by resentment. When the indigenous population's resentment explodes out of the confines of its "natural" passivity, they transgress the "scientific basis" of their inferiority: "...entonces el indio se levanta, olvida su manifiesta inferioridad, pierde el instinto de conservación y, oyendo a su alma repleta de odios, desfoga sus pasiones y roba, mata, asesina con saña atroz" (41). This pathological process which "sickens" the nation is traceable, on the one hand, to innate, psychological defects of the Indian, and, on the other, to historically acquired and internalized psychological defects resulting from his mistreatment by non-Indian society. Arguedas infers that without reform, this is a pathological pattern which is likely to recur.[34]

When combined with what Arguedas characterizes as the national megalomania of the mestizo, the innate passivity of the indigenous population leads to their exploitation by governmental officials and private speculators. Arguedas denotes this abuse with the colonial term of Indian administration, *caciquismo*: "Las explotaciones de quienes ejercen algún cargo, son de otra índole. El caciquismo, ha de verse en su lugar, es una de las más singulares manifestaciones de la enfermedad colectiva" (44). For Arguedas these local autocrats or *caciques* hold the Indians in complete contempt and view them as instruments for their own self-aggrandizement.

Yet even this historical degradation of the Indian is grounded in a pre-columbian source of indigenous degeneration. According to Arguedas the civil wars that plagued the Incan empire before the arrival of the Spanish had a debilitating effect on the race. Arguedas analyzes the results of these conflicts from a decidedly modern and Western point of view which privileges the autonomy of the individual. He alleges that the lack of individual autonomy within the Incan empire, along with an overly abundant natural wealth and

---

[34] But the term "reform" is used advisedly with regard to Arguedas. Arguedas' vision of reform was not to change the social system but to make those who work within it, whether they be landowners or peasants, fulfill their role in a moral fashion. This model for moral improvement was thwarted by his own linking of morality to race. Hence the pessimism of *Pueblo enfermo.*

easy, if not lazy existence, sowed the seeds of future decadence. The race "se moldeó a la pasividad," its collective personality is one of "obediencia pasiva," leaving it with an "alma femenina y dulce" which is "vegetal sin duda." This is the psychological profile which enables the conquistadors to conquer, enslave and exhaust the Indian. Through this contact with the egocentric, violent Spaniard of the Black Legend, the "weak" indigenous race exaggerates the defensive vices of its "feminine" psychological aspect. In this way, Arguedas argues, the now congenitally degenerate state of the Indian amounts to a Lamarckian or acquired evolutionary trait: "Entonces, ante la brutalidad del blanco, busca como toda raza débil su defensa en los vicios femeninos de la mentira, de la hipocresía, la disimulación y el engaño. Pero estos mismos vicios no son innatos a la raza. Los ha adquirido por contagio" (51). But this infection is genetically transmitted by those Indians saved by their "feminine vices," initiating what Arguedas characterizes as an inversion of natural selection.

Much more than the Indian, the real object of Arguedas' scorn in *Pueblo enfermo* is the *cholo*. Basically, *"cholo"* is a pejorative term for mestizo, but as the following passage from *Pueblo enfermo* suggests, the definition of the *cholo* is not that simple: "El *cholo* (raza mestiza) en cuanto se encumbra en su medio y ya es *señor*, y, por lo tanto, pertenece a la raza blanca" (32). The *cholo* is a mestizo who aspires to the social and racial position and privilege of the socially and empirically determined whiteness of the creole elite. Thus, strictly speaking, the *cholo* is not a biological category but a cultural product of transculturation. [35] But as the phrase in parenthesis "(raza mestiza)" in the above cited definition indicates, Arguedas does not make such fine distinctions between social and racial definitions. As we shall see, Arguedas uses the term *cholo* to criticize at the same time alleged racial, social and class faults. In this sense the term takes on a generic meaning of "corrupt," with its racial implications remaining as an unstated given.

Arguedas' first and most damning point of attack against the *cholo* is biological. His first reference to the long-standing debate on the health or degeneracy of mixed species or sub-species is made

---

[35] As Albarracín Millán states: "El 'cholo' tampoco es el mestizo, en sí, porque éste es una categoría étnica y aquél una de sus raíces culturales. En los hechos el 'cholo' es un fenómeno de transculturación que obedece a patrones raciales" (193).

in a passing allusion to studies which had investigated "hybridism and its fatal consequences." The choice of the terminology of hybridism is not in itself arbitrary. In fact, any term used to label people of "mixed" heritage (the notion of "mixed" itself being a constructed metaphor) invariably activates negative or positive scientific associations. The notion of the racial hybrid comes out of an appropriation of an internal debate within botany concerning the vitality and fecundity of plant hybrids. When biologists projected this discussion onto human beings the results were polemical and often pessimistic. Some followers of the "hybrid" model felt that such crossings among human beings were doomed to infertility, and thus eventual extinction, their favorite model being that of the mule. Others, such as Darwin, knew that there were obvious examples of cross-breading among different species but at the same time felt that natural selection would lead to sterility in the initial generation (Stepan 111). Others maintained the notion of partial fertility and degeneration among "hybrid" breeds.

One of the principal theoretical sources for Arguedas' characterization of the hybridism of the *cholo* was Le Bon. The gist of this French psychologist's position held that the offspring of racial cross-breeding were always inferior to the parent's "pure" racial character. Hybrids, Le Bon argued, were afflicted by congenital deficiencies of morality and integrity. For Le Bon, this inherently immoral and dissembling character made hybrid peoples wholly unsuitable to positions of power and authority. Moreover, this supposed innate corruption had larger implications for the political system inasmuch as it allegedly rendered hybrid populations unsuitable subjects for a popularly elected, democratic government. For Latin Americans, Le Bon's damning assessment of hybridity undercut the uniformity of national character deemed necessary for the development of their new republics. Le Bon made this point unequivocally in *The Psychology of Peoples*: "The first effect of inbreeding between different races is to destroy the soul of the races, and by their soul we mean that congeries of common ideas and sentiments which make the strength of peoples, and without which there is no such thing as a nation or a fatherland" (54).

For Arguedas, Le Bon's argument served to give scientific legitimacy and discursive modernity to historically established patterns of racial identity and discrimination already present in Latin America. In the nineteenth century, author-statesmen such as Sarmiento and Alberdi (and as we have seen at the turn-of-the-century their fellow Argentinean and precursor to Arguedas, Bunge) had stated that the hybrid or mixed populations of Latin America constituted the most serious and ingrained obstacles to economic development, modernization and the rationalization of the state. Arguedas, like Bunge before him, saw this as a pan-American problem:

> El *cholo* de Bolivia, Perú y Colombia, el *roto* de Chile, el *gaucho* de la Argentina y del Uruguay, etc., son una clase de gentes híbridas, sometidas a lentos procesos de selección, pero que todavía no han alcanzado a eliminar de sí las taras de su estirpe porque el problema de su modificación aun (*sic*) permanece latente en muchos países, siendo ese (*sic*), por su magnitud, la primordial labor educativa. (61)

In the context of Bolivia, Arguedas traces the nation's ills back to the defective psychology of the *cholo*. Obviously following the model established in Le Bon and Bunge's *Nuestra América*, Arguedas affirms that the *cholo* has received the worst traits from both of his parents' races. From the Spaniard he is afflicted with megalomania, aggressiveness and excessive rhetoric, whereas his indigenous ancestor has infected him with passivity, dependency, indifference and the "feminine" vices of lying, deceit and hypocrisy. The *cholo* is thus deemed to be a moral idiot, a reiteration of the scientific prejudice that women, children and all so-called inferior races are soul-less, immoral beings.

This permanent, youthful, degenerate and un-evolving state is linked by Arguedas to the very etiology of the word *cholo*. Based on the account of an unnamed colonial "cronista altoperuano," Arguedas attributes the origin of the term to the custom of a Spanish nobleman, who, after spending considerable time in Italy, addressed the mestizo in Italian as *fanicullo* or "jovencito" in Spanish, young man. This origin, Arguedas states, instilled in the *cholo* the anxiety, allied to a form of Nietzschean resentment, to vindicate his power and virility through ostentation and deception.

Significantly, the core of Arguedas' examination of the *cholo*'s supposed inferiority is class-based as well as race-. Arguedas' critique of the mestizo population is based on an analogy between racial mixing and social mobility. The *cholo* is the "social climber" *par excellence*. Arguedas is not alone in this belief. As Sander

Gilman has affirmed, for nineteenth-century degeneracy theorists such as Morel and Gobineau, the threat of social mobility was as great as the one posed by hybridization ("Sexology" 77).

The class analysis of *cholo* psychology assumes two fronts, a critique of the mestizo middle class of government bureaucrats and an accompanying analysis of the mestizo popular classes. The criticism of the *cholo* professional class is particularly important insofar as it is said to be leading the nation into decline. The main problem for Arguedas is the congenital lack of morality which makes *cholo* politicians, diplomats, military officials, lawyers and priests incapable of determining the morality of an action or policy. In the absence of this moral guidance they follow their own immediate self-interest or, as in the case of politicians, what Arguedas classifies (citing Nietzsche) as a biological herd instinct. Underlying the allegations of the professional middle class *cholo*'s pathology is his supposedly uncontrollable tendency to lie and simulate:

> El cholo abogado prefiere de las leyes aquellas que en su interpretación pueden torcer la justicia de una causa; el cholo político es falso e inestable en sus principios ordinarios, cuando los tiene; y el cholo legislador apenas sabe copiar leyes y disposiciones exóticas suponiendo ser labor fácil trocar el espíritu de las gentes para obligarles a proceder adaptándose a reglas contrarias a la íntima modalidad de su temperamento étnico. (61)

Arguedas make it blatantly clear that his criticism of the *cholo* is in effect an attack on the underdevelopment, or what he interprets as the inefficiency and corruption, of the Latin American middle class in general. He states that to discard these ills as pertaining only to Bolivians is to "desconocer con malicia las tendencias de la clase media de los demás países hispanoamericanos, donde, igualmente, se presenta como una clase manifiestamente inferior..." (61).

The examination of the mestizo masses is far less developed in the chapter on *cholo* psychology. The points of Arguedas' attack on the Bolivian masses is that they are lazy, prone to drink, and vulnerable to what he characterizes as barbaric, egalitarian political philosophies.[36] The larger, although indirect profile of the mestizo

---

[36] For Arguedas, such egalitarian political philosophies are not only "barbaric," they are unnatural. Here Arguedas is adhering to the tradition of "scientific" challenge to democracy and revolution initiated by critics of the French Revolution such as Hippolyte Taine, and later developed by Le Bon and Lombroso.

masses occurs in the chapter on the history of *caudillismo* in Bolivia, "De la sangre y el lodo en nuestra historia." Here the debilitating effects of ongoing civil wars are impugned to the degenerate
psychology of the mestizo *caudillos* and their mixed-race women
and followers. The masses who support these regional leaders are
referred to as a "multitud desenfrenada," "la turba" and "chusma."
Arguedas affirms, quoting none other than the father of Latin
American independence, Simón Bolívar, that the mestizo masses'
ascension to power through the *caudillos* is a reversal of evolution:
"Si fuera posible que una parte del mundo volviera al caos primitivo, este sería el último período de América" (179).

The case of the *caudillo* Daza is offered as an example of what
happens when the mestizo masses come to power. Daza falls from
power in a chaotic fashion, Arguedas alleges, because of his racial
shortcomings: "...sobre todo era cholo; tenía carne y espíritu de
plebe y sólo le preocupaban los afanes y las satisfacciones de momento, ... la satisfacción de sus enormes exigencias corporales; hol-
gar, beber, embriagarse, gastar mujeres, lucirse uniformes vis-
tosos..." (207). Daza embodies all of the so-called degenerative
traits of racial mixing: laziness, drunkenness, sexual promiscuity
and ostentatious megalomania.

It is not a coincidence that the section on white creole psychology should occur at the end of the chapter on mestizo psychology,
with its brevity and function suggesting a critical epilogue to mestizo predominance in Bolivian society. The scarcity of analysis of
white culture follows from Arguedas' lament about the scarcity of
"pure" white blood in Bolivia. For Arguedas even those who have
the social imprimatur of being white are subject to racial and environmental degeneration in the Americas. The racial faults of Bolivian whites are linked to the deficiencies of the Spanish race.
Whereas Arguedas definitely finds Spaniards to be the superior element in the Bolivian racial economy, he nevertheless borrows from
Bunge's in-depth assessment of Spain's relative racial inferiority in
comparison with Anglo-Saxon Europe. This denigration of the
Spanish heritage reiterates the findings of Spanish diagnosticians
of national infirmity such as Picavea and Ganivet. Spaniards are,
Arguedas maintains, inclined to aggressiveness, compulsiveness,
aboulia and dependency on governmental service, a disorder
Arguedas classifies as "empleomanía." Furthermore, Arguedas
states, Bolivians who have maintained a predominance of Spanish

"blood" are constantly under the threat of racial mixing and environmental degeneration. The threat is derived from the belief, noted earlier in relation to the urbanized Indian, that races degenerate when removed from their original environment. [37] Arguedas voices this belief when he offers the following summary of the fate of whites in Bolivia: "La hidalguía ha venido a menos, se ha mestizado, puede decirse. Se mantuvo todavía fuerte con las primeras generaciones y recién transplantada a tierras calientes de América" (63).

AMERICA THE "YOUNG" OR AMERICA THE "SICK"?

In the foreword to the third 1937 edition of *Pueblo enfermo*, Arguedas reflects, albeit indirectly, on the polemic surrounding its original publication in Latin America in 1909. For many Latin American intellectuals of the period, the multiple national infirmities diagnosed by Arguedas in *Pueblo enfermo* were not indicative of an alleged, permanent, congenital inferiority of Latin Americans, but rather, were attributable to the developmental deficiencies or childhood diseases of youthful nations and peoples.

As discussed earlier, this developmental view of Latin American nations was championed by Rodó in *Ariel*. Rodó communicated this vision of Latin America to Arguedas in a letter he wrote after reading *Pueblo enfermo*. He wrote:

> Usted titula su libro: *PUEBLO ENFERMO.* Yo lo titularía: *Pueblo niño.* Es concepto más amplio y justo quizás, y no excluye, sino que, en cierto modo, incluye al otro; porque la primera infancia tiene enfermedades propias y peculiares, cuyo más eficaz remedio radica en la propia fuerza de la vida, nueva y pujante, para saltar sobre los obstáculos que se le oponen.

It is significant that Arguedas included the gist of this letter in the foreword to the text's third edition. At a first glance we have

---

[37] Nancy Stepan has described this belief at some length. Regarding the scientific suspicion of "degenerate" colonial Europeans in the peripheries, she states: "Contrariwise, the 'proper' place of the white race was now defined as the temperate, 'civilized' Europe. When the white race moved out of its 'natural' home, it too underwent a process of biological degeneration, it became 'tropicalized'" (99).

two methodologically disparate works; Rodó's intentionally mythological, aesthetic and parabolic *Ariel*, as opposed to Arguedas' scientific, anthropological and *costumbrista Pueblo enfermo*. The common ground underlying these and other national essays of turn-of-the-century Latin America is the concern for "national" self-examination and definition. More profound than this commonality of intention, however, is the intersection of various figurative discourses basic to the very concept of the Americas and the Americans. The deliberate conjoining of two apparently different or antagonistic images of America, of America as "sick" along with America as "young," occurs within the wider conceptual frame of organicist thought which conceives of the nation as an organism subject to vicissitudes of good and/or ill health. In this sense what is interesting about Rodó's amendment to *Pueblo enfermo* is that he does *not* dispute the diagnosis of illness, but its proper classification. For Rodó the symptoms described by Arguedas do not entail a terminally ill patient or nation, but rather constitute the growing pains and illnesses of youth which can be outgrown through social evolution.

However, upon a close reading of the entire foreword to the 1937 edition, Arguedas' inclusion of Rodó's letter and his avowed self-correction in the light of Rodó's criticism appears to be more an act of self-reaffirmation or defiance than contrition. Immediately after admitting that of all the objections made to *Pueblo enfermo*, "este de Rodó fué uno de los que más impresión me produjeron," Arguedas goes on to refute the hypothesis of Latin America as a set of normally evolving, young nations and reiterates his original claim that this evolution is impeded by Latin America's psycho-biological inferiority. For Arguedas, "youth" is, and will always be, the prominent feature of Latin America, because, for him, it is a racial, and not a developmental issue: "sus primitivos elementos étnicos," as he puts it, prevent Latin America from adapting to the conditions of modernity.

Nevertheless, Arguedas pays homage to Rodó, stating that his recommendations "han producido, pues, su fruto." Yet this image of fruit proves to be problematic within the foreword to *Pueblo enfermo* as well as within the greater rhetorical imagery of Arguedas' writings. Shortly after praising Rodó, whom he refers to in *Pueblo enfermo* as "este mentor de la juventud americana" (243), the very term of his praise is undermined. The positive effects of Rodó's recommendations, the "fruit," is given another, conflicting connotation. Whereas the fruit produced by Rodó's suggestions connotes youthful, fresh produce, the usage subsequently employed by Arguedas in the next section of the foreword conjures up an antagonistic image of sickly or rotten fruit.

Arguedas presents this conflicting fruit imagery in the defense of *Pueblo enfermo* against its detractors. The purpose of the book was, Arguedas affirms, to describe the nation as it was: "presentándolo como inhábil, enfermo de veras y muy gravemente al lado de otros que mostraban entonces faz robusta y limpia, aunque como ciertos frutos, llevasen dentro la hedionda podre y el gusano vil. Y todos eran, poco más o menos, *Pueblos Enfermos...*" (X). In this passage not only does Arguedas proclaim the allegedly obvious sickness of his own native Bolivia, but also goes on to question the apparently healthy condition of other Latin American states as well. Latin American nations, pictured here as fruit, including those which are apparently healthy, "que mostraban entonces faz robusta y limpia," may conceal the enervating worm of internal corruption.

This graphic image of Latin American youth and nationality as prematurely rotten fruit seems to have been productive for Arguedas. In a political "Manifiesto" written three years after the foreword to the 1937 edition of *Pueblo enfermo*, he utilizes a similar language to condemn the decadent youth of Bolivia's upper class:

> Tampoco soy enemigo de la juventud. Lo que tampoco puedo disculpar y de lo que me muestro francamente enemigo es de los mozalbetes audaces, inescrupulosos, arrivistas, cínicos y conveniencieros. Son frutos podridos en verde y de ellos no se puede esperar nada. (Díaz Arguedas 17)

Returning to the foreword to the 1937 edition of *Pueblo enfermo*, the sincerity of Arguedas' incorporation of Rodó's argument would seem thus to be in doubt. Specifically, after comparing Rodó's influence to fruit, Arguedas goes on to challenge the purity of all fruit regardless of appearance. This apparent slight to Rodó is further evidenced by the vehemently defiant ending of the foreword, in which Arguedas lashes out at Rodó-like optimism, denouncing it as "el fácil optimismo de los satisfechos, era la verdadera mentira; que los entusiastas de la raza y los propaladores de las virtudes, méritos y cualidades del pueblo boliviano eran simples voceadores de frases de circunstancia para ganar electores, adquirir el título de patriotas y ocupar un sitio de privilegio en el casillero de los más altos puestos públicos..." (XI).

Before entering into the immediate turn-of-the-century circumstances which inform texts such as *Pueblo enfermo*, it is necessary to briefly review the history of the oppositional or complimentary discourses of "America the young" or "America the sick". For although the emphasis of this study will be on nineteenth-century developments in the natural and social sciences and their relation to the discourse of identity in Latin America, it is obvious, yet necessary, to state that other pre-scientific or differently conceived, "proto-scientific" discourses preceded those of the eighteenth and nineteenth centuries.

In the nineteenth century the polemic surrounding the alleged youth, immaturity and/or biological weakness of Latin America was inscribed into the historical obsession with the medicalization of sexuality characteristic of the period. This preoccupation with the sexual followed from the new configuration of social alliances governing marriage, the transmission of property and the distribution of social power within the modern bourgeois family and the liberal capitalist state. The nineteenth-century sexologist Krafft-Ebing emphasized this collaboration between physicians and the state in the monitoring of sexuality for the public good: "Inasmuch as the preservation of chastity and morals is one of the most important reasons for the existence of the commonwealth, the state cannot be too careful, as a protector of morality, in the struggle against sensuality" (498).

Of principal concern to this reconfiguration of sexual economy was the vigilance over and disciplining of female and infantile sexualities. To better understand this fixation with childhood sexuality it is necessary to quote from Michel Foucault's *The History of Sexuality* at some length:

> 2. *A pedagogization of children's sex:* a double assertion that practically all children indulge or are prone to indulge in sexual activity; and that, being unwarranted, at the same time, "natural" and "contrary to nature," this sexual activity posed physical and moral, individual and collective dangers; children were defined as "preliminary" sexual beings, on this side of sex, yet within it, astride a dangerous dividing line. Parents, families, educators, doctors, and eventually psychologists would have to take charge,

in a continuous way, of this precious and perilous, dangerous and endangered sexual potential: this pedagogization was especially evident in the war against onanism, which in the West lasted nearly two centuries. (104)

This obsession with juvenile sexuality, chastity and morality is central to the Latin American essays under discussion here. Whereas in *Ariel*, Rodó takes an optimistically cheerful, yet anxiously repressive, position on juvenile sexuality, other Latin American author-pedagogues of the period are not as hopeful in their treatments of the subject.

In both *Nuestra América* (1903) and *La Educación* (1903) Bunge deals with the dissolute frivolity of Argentina's privileged youth. For Bunge, the problem of upper class youth is identical to the diagnosed deficiencies of creole psychology. This psychological profile contains the accumulated faults of Spanish, indigenous and African ancestry, what Bunge characterizes as a combination of laziness, sadness and arrogance (Terán 38). The only hope Bunge holds out for Argentina's elite youth is that they will, in effect, disappear and be replaced by harder-working, ethically driven immigrants; a belief Bunge asserts in this passage from *Nuestra América*:

> Felizmente, si su ejemplo y su influencia preponderan aún, mañana caerán, y de pronto, como piedra en el abismo. No sabiendo esos jóvenes pseudo-aristócratas conservar sus bienes, sus despilfarros les van dejando ya sin fortuna; sin fortuna merman de prestigio, mientras el elemento inmigratorio adquiere, para sustituirles, los bienes que ellos pierden y la cultura que nunca tuvieran... (158)

Agustín Álvarez is another Argentinean author who had considerable documentable influence on Arguedas. Álvarez takes up the issue of Latin American youth in his influential *Manual de patología política* (1899). Like Bunge, Álvarez criticizes the perennially spoiled and infantile behavior of Argentina's youth. On one level Álvarez attributes this adolescent dissolution to the child-rearing practices of Argentina's bourgeoisie. Álvarez blames Argentine parents for spoiling, coddling and over-protecting their children. The Argentine father is found to be too lenient: "rara vez castiga a sus hijos" (217). Yet for Álvarez, the real culprit in the corruption of

Argentine youth is the mother, who, despite her complete devotion, is by her psycho-physiological nature unable to instill a sense of social responsibility or independence in her over-indulged child. For Álvarez, the results of this undisciplined, dangerously permissive upbringing are disastrous for the Argentine national character inasmuch as they debilitate the population in both mind and body:

> Como plantas de invernáculo resultamos débiles de físico por exceso de cuidados y algodones, y tísicos de alma por exceso de indulgencia. Porque nos han privado de la represión paterna que cura y no ofende, nos sobreviene fuera del nido la represión de los extraños que ofende y no cura: cuando pitos flautas, cuando flautas pitos. (217-218)

Álvarez completes this *costumbrista* sketch of the defects of the Argentinean family with medical and psychological warnings concerning lax morals and premature sexual activity among the young:

> El joven ignora que no hay peor pérdida de fuerzas, que tales comercios abaten el ánimo, que después de 10 años de semejante vida habrá perdido *la mitad de su voluntad*, que sus pensamientos tendrán un dejo de amargura y de tristeza, que sus resortes interiores se habrán relajado o doblegado. (*sic* 321)

The prognosis given here, supported by an excerpt from a letter by "El doctor Antonio Arraga, el distinguido especialista en enfermedades de los niños" (321), is reminiscent of the figure of the chronic masturbator of eighteenth and nineteenth-century sexology or Ganivet's abulic personality in the *Idearium español*. Given the shared philosophical-medical sources of Ganivet and Álvarez, Hippolyte Taine and Théodule Ribot, this should not be surprising.

Individual pathology leads, as the title of Álvarez's *Manual* suggests, to collective social or "political" pathology. How, Álvarez wonders, will the future military and political leaders of Latin America acquire the moral discipline, independence of mind and strength of body and spirit necessary to fulfill their functions in a society and culture which produces such degenerate youth? Concerned with the fate of democracy, Álvarez questions the voting sensibilities of a dissolute youth which has systematically participated in immoral if not illicit behavior, who "a la edad electoral ya han practicado con éxito una buena parte del código penal" (320).

Within the context of Argentina, Álvarez believes that the problem of degenerate youth can be addressed and completely resolved. In his educational optimism he is quite distant from the racially determinist pessimism of Bunge, and, as we shall see, Arguedas. Álvarez argues that the Argentinean model for child-rearing must be discarded in favor of what he describes as the North American model. On this point his difference from promoters of a decidedly "hellenized" cultural and scholastic model, such as Rodó, is quite striking. What Rodó sees as crass utilitarianism, Álvarez idealizes as pragmatic discipline. Álvarez exhorts Argentina to emulate the North American practice of expecting and requiring disciplined "adult" behavior of children before they are in fact adults. In this way, Álvarez argues, North American youth is prepared to accept the freedom and responsibility of adulthood when they come of age, unlike the "patriarchically raised" Argentine youth who await and prepare for adulthood in "el club o el café" (323).

In *Pueblo enfermo*, we witness the influence of Bunge's and Álvarez's ideas about the congenital and/or acquired weakness of Latin America's youth combined with residues of the previous colonial stereotypes of the "young" topography and peoples of America, particularly in Arguedas' criticism of Bolivian university students, a criticism deeply embedded in his own personal recollections of his student years.

In this account Arguedas states that his fellow students were lazy and decadent sorts who could only manage to read extremely short books which would not conflict with their "espíritu rutinario y perezoso de los universitarios de ese tiempo, a nuestros inveterados hábitos de pereza, holganza y disipación" (111). To some extent this description of juvenile enervation is itself a subject of Arguedas' own literary studies or readings, in this way blending his sense of a lived reality together with an ideologically fictional and constructed discourse of youthful degeneration. Arguedas reflected upon the mediating effects of this Spanish literary model for the construction of his own sense of Bolivian youthful decadence in the following way: "Y al fin obraban las fuerzas del mal y el estudiante boliviano era la reproducción fiel y exacta del modelo que se ofrecía por la misma época en España, según esa curiosa y puntual pintura hecha por Ricardo Macías Picavea, muerto en 1899" (111).

This deplorable state of Bolivia's youth, according to Arguedas, can be traced to causes strikingly similar to those described by

Álvarez. Like Álvarez, Arguedas attributes the youthful decadence of the creole elite to an unhealthy family atmosphere and inadequate cultural practices. In brief, it is a deficiency of education and upbringing which is diagnosed by Arguedas in a sort of "*costumbrismo* of ills" narrative.

As with Álvarez, the Latin American mother is for Arguedas a central malefactor in the corruption of Latin American youth. Chapter VIII of *Pueblo enfermo*, "La mujer boliviana. Su rol social," describes how elite creole women suffer from an absolute lack of education and a sentimentally disfigured understanding of religion and existence which restrict them to an idle and pointless life of gossip and material acquisitiveness. Accordingly, the creole woman lacks ambition for learning or social responsibilities and lives:

> según su deseo, y por eso la mujer boliviana, salvo, naturalmente, excepciones, a pesar de su alta penetración de espíritu, poco se preocupa de adaptarse a la corriente intelectual de una sociedad para imponer en ella su dominio efectivo y durable... de manera que aun trayendo cierta superficial cultura de los centros de enseñanza, primitivos y superficiales, se pierde y extingue ésta con el diario trajeteo absolutamente inintelectual, frívolo y poco expansivo. (148)[38]

Given this negative view of the elite creole woman's mental and spiritual faculties, she becomes an easy scapegoat for the alleged decadence of Bolivian youth. In short, Arguedas alleges that she is an unfit mother, lacking a sense of morality: "la mujer boliviana, la americana más bien," Arguedas affirms, "no está preparada para desempeñar dicho rol" (153). Significantly, very much unlike Álvarez's accompanying critique of the failure of paternal guidance and discipline, Arguedas is silent on this point.

Arguedas asserts that Bolivian youth, raised in this vacuum of morality and social responsibility, specifically male youth, engages in the vices of smoking, drinking, gamboling and whoring. The results of this dissolute life are similar to those predicted in Álvarez's

---

[38] It is interesting to note that the woman of the oligarchical elite is generically referred to as "la mujer boliviana" while women of other socio-ethnic categories are denominated as "la mujer indígena" or those of "procedencia mestiza," all of which are ascribed their own psychological profiles, social roles, and debilities.

Manual de patología política. Namely, such unscrupulous pastimes produce that paradoxical figure of degeneracy theory, the aged youth, the youthful dotard who has brought on his premature degeneration through moral transgression, substance abuse and sexual over-indulgence: "A los veinticinco años es ya hombre gastado, marchito, envejecido" (153). Thus what is diagnosed as a lack of cultural and familial discipline, or "sick" national customs, results in the psychologically and physiologically damaging effects of energy depletion and degeneration. More importantly for the nation, these individually acquired debilities and vices can be genetically stored and transmitted in the "Lamarckian" fashion we have noted before to future generations, constituting a veritable threat to national virility and health.

Although Arguedas puts much of the blame for this state of affairs on a lack of social responsibility and discipline, a culturally and socially, though not necessarily politically conservative position, he also signals sexual segregation as a cause of national degeneration. Here Arguedas assumes the discourse of a liberal, social reformer attempting to bring modernity to his native Bolivia. According to Arguedas, the segregation of the sexes is to the detriment of both genders. He determines that this separation is especially harmful for boys, causing them to form excessively strong ties among themselves, forcing them to become men without having experienced the mollifying and enchanting effects of "la convivencia femenina" (154). Instead of a healthy and chaste education, Arguedas laments that parents leave their children's fate in the hands of "profesores incompetentes" who administer an anti-social, sexually segregated education. Ironically, perhaps, the exclusively male to male relationships between students and mentor portrayed in *Ariel* as a source of regeneration are viewed precisely as a source of national enervation and decline in *Pueblo enfermo*.

Artificially separated, Arguedas explains, the sexes reach the age "where nature imposes its responsibilities." The combination of natural desire and absolute separation leads to the psychological and physiological calamity of premature marriage. Both men and women come to marriage ill prepared and improperly socialized for such a union. Young men, Arguedas affirms, arrive at their wedding day in a state of premature dissolution as a result of their exclusively male education and practices: "Lleva el hombre una naturaleza gastada, hábitos viciosos, carácter despótico, voluntad indomable y

ardiente de conocer prácticamente todos los misterios del amor..."
(154). According to Arguedas, young women are also ill equipped
for these unions. They approach marriage in a haze of "supersti-
tions" and "fanaticisms" instilled in them by their poor education.

Married under these unhealthy circumstances, Bolivian youth
are unable to understand one another, meet one another's needs,
much less fulfill social responsibilities. It is this last failure, what Arguedas terms as the inability to grasp the "trascendencia social" of
marriage, the young couple's "absoluta ignorancia de deberes y
obligaciones" (155), which he finds so detrimental to the nation.

At the root of Arguedas' preoccupation with marriage is a
greater underlying concern with the family as an allegorical microcosm for the national. In this sense, we can read Arguedas' account
of the ills of marriage among Bolivia's elite youth as a variant of the
pattern of narrative romance which, as Doris Sommer points out,
links biological reproduction to national production, growth and
consolidation: "Part of the conjugal romance's national project, perhaps the main part, is to produce legitimate citizens, literally to engender civilization" (86).

This is the ultimate failure of the premature weddings denounced by Arguedas in *Pueblo enfermo*. Not only do these unhappy marriages represent a tragedy for the couple involved, but also
for the nation. Lacking in mutual affection and desire, the couple
cannot, as Sommer observes, produce legitimate, healthy citizens.
The requirement for reciprocal desire in procreation is a decidedly
Latin American injunction against non-reproductive sexual practices and the violent history of "unrequited" love and rape associated with social-erotic relations of power during the conquest and
colonization of Latin America (Sommer 87).

This historically ingrained insistence on reciprocal love and desire in Latin American literature was reinforced by philosophical
and scientific beliefs of the late nineteenth to early twentieth centuries. This idea, referred to as "impression" in Otto Weininger's
Sex and Character, affirms that the offspring of an ideally untrue or
infelicitous sexual union is mentally and/or physically inferior or
degenerate. The violence of rape or the indifference of the "marriage of convenience" manifest themselves in organically inferior
children.

These accumulated historical and scientific concerns regarding
the inharmonious nature of Bolivia's young married couples lead

Arguedas to characterize the children produced by these unions as congenitally degenerate:

> De matrimonios así prematuramente concebidos y más prematu-
> ramente llevados a cabo, ha nacido toda una generación enfer-
> ma, las engendradas por ésta traen marcada decrepitud, y así,
> lentamente, sucesivamente se va extinguiendo la virilidad de la
> raza, condición preciosa de la vida de un pueblo, y cayendo en la
> fatiga física, que es la que menos debía de sentir, porque es pro-
> pio de pueblos que han vivido bastante y en su vida sufrido
> grandes trastornos y sobrellevado profundas crisis. (155)

In this passage the acquired vices and infirmities of the young Bo-livian male's upbringing combine with the organically damaging effects of an unreciprocally desired or inharmonious union, resulting in weakened offspring and a sickly nation. Significantly, the debilitation of the nation is once again grounded in the male body and psyche. The debilitation of the nation is equivalent to the dissipation of male fluids, energy and spirit, lumped together by Arguedas under the generic concept of "virilidad." In chapter XII of *Pueblo enfermo*, titled "Causas de esterilidad intelectual," Arguedas once again conflates notions of youth and organic deficiency in his discussion of Bolivian and Latin American cultural and political phenomena. In this instance the subject of his reflection is what he deems to be the lack of original, autonomous art in Bolivia.

In this chapter Arguedas slips back and forth between notions of a collective social and psychological immaturity and notions of individual and group pathology to account for the alleged literary shortcomings of Bolivia. The title of the chapter opens the discussion by invoking notions of disease or organic disfunction. What is promised by the title is an etiology, an investigation of the "causes" of the mental disease or disorder of "intellectual sterility." It is not clear whether this condition is an individual or group pathology.

Arguedas posits that the organic development of national literatures in Latin America requires the conservation and investigation of indigenous cultures, which he qualifies as "ya de algún desarrollo." Unfortunately, Arguedas laments, creole intellectuals are self-absorbed and too immersed in the socio-political neglect of the indigenous populations. That Arguedas took this criticism seriously is itself a matter of literary history. His novels *Pisagua* (1903), *Wata*

Wara (1904), *Vida Criolla* (1905) and *Raza de Bronce* (1923) were ground-breaking works in the investigation of Indian culture and in the foundation of indigenism as a literary movement. In fact it has been argued that the first version of *Pueblo enfermo*, possibly written in 1904, was contemporaneous with *Wata Wara* (Rodríguez-Luis 79). Nevertheless in this same chapter on intellectual "sterility" Arguedas blames the presence of Indian blood as a source of mental "atrophy" which impedes the development of a sense of the beautiful in contemporary Bolivia. Arguedas describes the indigenous aesthetic as one which defines the utilitarian as the beautiful, as in "un campo de patatas." For Arguedas, this utilitarian aesthetic sensibility is ultimately responsible for the Bolivian elite's lack of aesthetic appreciation, a deficit which resulted in the demolition of the ancient indigenous city of Tiahuanacu. Such mind-boggling zigzags of appreciation and contempt for Bolivia's autochthonous peoples are characteristic of *Pueblo enfermo*. As Juan Albarracín Millán states: "así el arguedismo pudo ser, al mismo tiempo, una apasionada condenación del indio y también iniciador del indigenismo en la literatura..." (55).

If he oscillated between admiration and disdain for indigenous peoples, Arguedas was absolutely negative in his condemnation of creole writers. The criticism Arguedas employs in his attack comes in undiluted form from one of degeneracy theory's most popular and influential promoters, Max Nordau.

Arguedas' description of creole writers repeats in particular the criticism Nordau had hurled at the Pre-Raphaelites: "Otra de las irremediables debilidades de nuestros autores criollos consiste en cultivar, esmerosa y amorosamente su *yo*" (242). For both Nordau and Arguedas, such egocentric writing constituted a puerile example of degenerate immaturity. Another psychological diagnosis which Arguedas borrows from Nordau in his examination of creole writing is the neurotic necessity to constantly form literary schools, movements and groups. Following Nordau, Arguedas asserts that this need for incessant group affiliation demonstrates a congenital inability for independent thinking and a childish need for constant infighting and gossip: "Se forman pequeños grupos, capillitas, que diría Nordau. Y es la vida de inquietudes eternas, llena de chismecillos, murmuraciones veladas, un continuo y agotador vaivén de malas pasiones incontenibles que ocupan toda la actividad y esterilizan los espíritus..." (242). The unstated but implicit assertion here is that this literary behavior approximates the negative caricature of elite feminine society, and is therefore entirely unsuitable for the virile project of establishing a national literature.

The diagnosis of Bolivian literary deficiencies in *Pueblo enfermo*, and the attribution of this inferiority to the organic and psychological inadequacies of Bolivian writers, closely resembles the discourse of enervation employed in the analysis of juvenile male degeneration in general. Arguedas repeats the connection we have noted before between the damaging effects of a dissolute lifestyle on a yet unformed mind and body and the loss of internal male energy. As Arguedas states: "mozos no aun formados" whose "resortes de vida interior" are qualified as "flojos," push themselves beyond their mental capacities. This process is one of masculine depletion which Arguedas compares with the physically "draining" activities of driving, sports and sex with prostitutes. Arguedas' diagnosis of literary decadence follows the formula used in his analysis of youth, premature marriage and degenerate offspring which began "A los veinticinco años...," only this time the age has gone up five years: "A los treinta años los escritores están vacíos, desinflados, porque o ya han dado todo lo que llevaban dentro, y era poco y malo, o los ha devorado el empleo que acabaron de alcanzar escribiendo..." (244). In this passage the youthful phallic power of Bolivian writers is, rather explicitly, squandered and "deflated."

In a critique that still resonates today for its debunking of a Eurocentric colonial imaginary, Arguedas criticizes Bolivian poets for imitating the physiological symbolism of beauty and the psychology of intimacy and sensuality found in nineteenth-century European literature: "Y así, loan v. gr., las cabelleras blondas y los ojos azules de sus amadas, de cuyos labios beben aromas y mieles, y no se percatan de que por las venas de sus amadas corre pura sangre mestiza y que sus cabelleras no son blondas sino negras, y no azules sus ojos, sino pardo o negros..." (245).

Arguedas also attributes the lack of a vigorous national literature to the violent history of civil war and "caudillaje" which preoccupied Bolivia in the nineteenth and early twentieth centuries. For Arguedas, such Bolivian literature has "anemic tonalities" which correspond to "abnormal states." But the abnormality he is referring to is spiritual, geographical and racial, as well as historical. He speaks of a general spiritual sterility, the monotony of the *pampa* and the spiritual poverty of the Indian soul. The distraction of this so-called abnormal history, combined with the internal deficiencies of the Bolivian authors, has, Arguedas claims, incapacitated them, preventing them from achieving what Arguedas defines as the responsibility of a national literature: "Su deber es desentrañar la psicología del grupo. La mejor obra literaria sería, por lo tanto, aquella que mejor ahonde el análisis del alma nacional y la presente en observación intensa, con todas sus múltiples variaciones" (246). Thus Arguedas' prescription for a national literature is that it be a clinical, psychological practice along the same medical model of *Pueblo enfermo*. In this sense the site of enunciation and the enunciation itself are identical. For Arguedas, however, the Bolivian author is too immature and degenerate, more of a patient than a doctor, to perform this function.

THE PATHOLOGY OF SIMULATION IN PUBLIC AND PRIVATE LIFE

> Simular es inventar o, mejor, aparentar y así eludir nuestra condición. La disimulación exige mayor sutileza: el que disimula no representa, sino que quiere hacer invisible, pasar desapercibido, sin renunciar a su ser. (38)

The issue of simulation, positively appraised by Octavio Paz in the above passage from *El laberinto de la soledad*, was also a central concern for Arguedas in *Pueblo enfermo*. But whereas Paz views simulation as a complicated, creative, existentialist break with representation and as an innovative attempt to redefine the self, Arguedas saw only self-deception, pathological lying and collective dementia in this desire to "eludir nuestra condición."

What Arguedas perceives as a deeply ingrained psychological propensity for simulation, pretense and deception in the Bolivian psyche is also classified as one of the principal causes of national decomposition. In this light we can observe how the themes of national self-deception and simulation recur throughout *Pueblo enfermo* in Arguedas' analysis of the political system, the press, the psychology of women, literature, race relations and Bolivian history. In fact this leitmotif of the peril of simulation serves to interrelate these specific compartmentalized critiques.

In some sense the notion of simulation in *Pueblo enfermo* is a softening or euphemism for two principal character faults which

Arguedas impugns to Bolivians: lying and ostentation. This euphemism grows out of the initial chapters of *Pueblo enfermo* on Indian and *cholo* psychology where Arguedas categorizes both groups as congenital liars, albeit for different reasons, and attributes the penchant for ostentation or "el boato" to the *cholo* population.

Inasmuch as Arguedas states that "La historia de Bolivia está escrita y hecha por los *cholos*," any abnormal personality traits associated with them can be expected to have an unhealthy effect upon the nation. The implicit understanding that Bolivian governmental, cultural and social institutions are run by *cholos* makes it redundant, at least for Arguedas, constantly to remind the reader that the *cholo* or *chola* psychological profile is the culprit.

Again following Bunge's assertion that the psychological derives from the physical in terms of geography and physiology, Arguedas links the national penchant for simulation to the dramatic geographic diversity of Bolivia. Arguedas sums up the disproportional relationship between Bolivia's topographic magnitude and what he believes to be its racial inferiority in the following sentence: "Todo es inmenso en Bolivia, todo, menos el hombre" (99). As a consequence of the geographic, botanical and zoological richness, Arguedas maintains, the Bolivian imagination can only conceive of grandeur and perfection. In this sense, he argues, Bolivians are determined visually. Surrounded by physical wealth and cut off from the rest of the world by their geographic isolation, Bolivians are said to be stuck in a psychological trap of self-valorization and ingrained indifference towards the outside world. It is a classic argument of positivist, psychological, geographical determinism of the kind made famous by Hippolyte Taine and others.

Arguedas employs the psychological disorder of megalomania, an illness characterized by delusions of grandeur and power, to characterize the state of the national psyche. Moreover, Arguedas goes on to state that this megalomaniac disorder is "común a todos los países indoamericanos," thereby combining racial along with geographic causalities. For Arguedas, the transparency or omnipresence of this megalomania masks the real conditions and problems that face Latin America and particularly Bolivia. In this sense Arguedas allows for both a voluntary and involuntary basis for the inclination for deception and simulation in Bolivia. But whether it is conscious or unconscious, the ubiquity of this megalomaniac simulation covers up the real, and perhaps central issue of *Pueblo enfer-*

mo, namely how to break with this collective delusion or conspiracy of grandeur and address what Arguedas views as a gap between Bolivia's exceedingly high self-esteem and its national corruption and underdevelopment. This leads Arguedas to state what he believes to be one of two possibilities: either the nation is not as wealthy in natural resources as everyone thinks or the nation is racially inferior and incapable of self-development:

> Y, una de dos: o esos países de la América Latina no son tan prodigiosamente ricos como se pregona siempre, o la raza que los puebla es raza en decadencia e inhábil para aceptar el progreso moderno porque casi todos esos nuestros países, unos más que otros, son pobres, carecen de grandes industrias, no disponen de capitales, ni hacen lujo de iniciativa y de espíritu emprendedor. (100)

Obviously for Arguedas this is merely a rhetorical choice since the whole of his *Pueblo enfermo* is dedicated to proving the second of the two possibilities. It is equally obvious that the choice offered by Arguedas is a false dichotomy which excludes the historical sources of Bolivia's poverty, namely its colonial exploitation at the hands of Spain and then its late nineteenth century insertion into the international market as a disempowered source of raw materials. In this sense Arguedas interprets the lack of tools necessary for facilitating modernization and industrialization in Bolivia such as an adequate system of roads, a modern mail and communications system, large amounts of readily available investment capital and the scientifically and mentally prepared managerial, entrepreneurial and technical classes capable of developing its abundant mineral wealth, not as the results of a protracted, centuries-long period of deliberate foreign underdevelopment and internal feudalism or *latifundismo*, but rather impugned this condition to internal racial debility. In this sense Arguedas' project of national introspection and analysis is a denial of the substantive causes of Bolivia's political and economic weakness.

For Arguedas, a principal manifestation of this megalomania is political simulation, or the farce of parliamentarian government in Bolivia. According to Arguedas, the Bolivian government consists of two groups: those who systematically oppose the government and those who unconditionally support it. Arguedas posits that the names and policies of these parties are of little importance inasmuch as they are exchangeable, changing with the period under the banner of liberals, republicans, conservatives, nationalists etc., a process confirmed by Edgar Ávila Echazú in his *Resumen y antología de la literatura boliviana*: "Pese a la aparente divergencia ideológica-política, conservadores y liberales gobiernan el país con los mismos fundamentos socio-económicos, y su alternabilidad en el poder no implicó ningún cambio básico de la estructura material de la nación" (85). Arguedas explains that despite their rhetorically adversarial nature the two parties, regardless of their name, share the same vice: demagoguery.

Just what constitutes the basis for the critique of this demagoguery is of great importance for the consideration of Arguedas' ideological position concerning race and politics in Bolivia. Juan Albarracín Millán has argued that *Pueblo enfermo* was written as an indictment of the political corruption of the supposedly prosperous liberal administration of Montes, and that the ensuing counterattacks of the government and the liberal press managed to stain Arguedas with the stigma of racism and unpatriotic thinking (187). In this way, Albarracín Millán argues, the vehemently conservative, racist and corrupt officials and press allies have been fundamental in establishing the historically negative reception of *Pueblo enfermo*. According to this logic the main thrust of Arguedas' critique of the Montes' regime is moral and not racist or "anti-Bolivian." Whereas Albarracín Millán is certainly right to point out the extreme hypocrisy and moral vacancy of many of Arguedas' contemporary critics, to state that the text was solely an indictment of political corruption and simulation misses the point.

To better understand Arguedas' critique of political demagoguery and deception, it is necessary to consider the specific ills he perceived within the body politic of Bolivia. The object of Arguedas' condemnation was excessive political rhetoric which glossed over the real problems of the country and created its own self-congratulating and sustaining verbal reality. The terms Arguedas uses to describe this extravagant oratory come out of clinical psychology and medicine. He refers to this uncontrollable need to utter political gibberish as "onomatomanía" and "verbomanía," organic mental disorders or manias. The description of this political charade, here characterized as a disorder, is not grounded in the language of political corruption, power or privilege but rather in terms of a clinical diagnosis:

...es la onomatomanía en grado agudo, el furor incontenible de alinear palabras y frases sin sentido. Concíbese que en un momento de exaltación verbal pueda llegarse a la incorrección de la frase, pero no la absoluta ausencia de lógica. Un orador exaltable atacado de delirio en plena peroración hablaría con más cordura. (103)

Arguedas' pathological construction of political rhetoric may well have been influenced by his readings of Bunge and Álvarez. In *Nuestra América* Bunge classifies the politician's uncontrollable propensity to engage in over-abundant political rhetoric as "parlamentaritis":

Hay que curar al *criollo* de su parlamentaritis, mórbida peste mental, crónica y aguda, consistente en una histérica pasión por los discursos kilométricos, por las reformas architrascendentales, por la contienda parlamentaria con todas sus vanas fórmulas de "hago moción", "como dice el ilustrado colega", "los que estén por la afirmativa", etc., etc. (167)

Bunge's diagnosis differs from Arguedas' medicalizations of political behavior in that the former's term suggests both biological disease, denoted by the suffix -*itis*, and a mental dysfunction or disorder, hysteria. Moreover, Bunge's description of political pathology is interesting in that it links the alleged biological and mental illness of creole politicians with a specific form of government. In this sense it is important to point out that Bunge's term for political illness does not in itself indicate a pathology of speaking, like Arguedas' "verbomanía" or "onomatomanía," but rather signals the form of government as the origin of the problem. Hence, for Bunge, "parlamentaritis" is not merely the affliction of specific deficient individual politicians within an otherwise functioning system, but rather a sick form of government in itself. The parliamentary process of inter-party negotiation and conflict, as well as social reforms, are as pathological as the inherent mental faults of the creole politicians themselves.

The immediate Latin American precursor for both Bunge and Arguedas in the taxonomy of political illness is Agustín Álvarez. In his *Manual de patología política* Álvarez makes visible the connections between individual neuropathological dysfunction, speech disorders, the pathology of specific parliamentary procedures and the greater theme of simulation or illusion as the source of national decline and illness as elaborated by Arguedas in *Pueblo enfermo*. Álvarez states that the sickness affecting political life in Argentina is analogous to that which afflicts society. Society's attempts to cure the political sickness, Álvarez affirms, are doomed to failure unless society cures itself first. In this way Álvarez compares political reform to the ineffective treatment of the superficial symptoms of a disease. Accordingly, mere political reform exacerbates the condition, creating the illusion that the patient or nation is well, thus allowing the real cause of illness to fester. The primary instrument of this unhealthy reformist therapy is political oratory. Quoting the degeneracy theorist Théodule Ribot, Álvarez states that rhetorical dementia of politicians is a neurological disorder: "Se ha notado, dice Ribot, que las lesiones de la primera y segunda circunvolución frontal debilitan la voluntad y que entonces se exagera la habladuría; disminuye la ejecución y aumentan los planes vanos" (42). Following Álvarez's argument, Argentina's politically and organically debilitating governmental procedures and reforms, which he lists as "La manía de hacer reglamentos," "la manía de hacer comisiones," and "la capacidad para confeccionarlos," are naturally articulated within the individual and parliamentary political mind with a frequency that is inversely proportional to the ability to realize them.

For Arguedas, the danger posed by the political speech pathologies of Bolivian politicians clearly goes beyond the confines of the governing elite. This insipid rhetoric obscures the genuine problems of the nation and, what is worse, it is contagious. Arguedas states that far from being critical of political oratory, the masses enjoy and are easily duped by it. Thus the disease is neither cured nor even contained, threatening to "convertirse en endémico e incurable" (103). The sources of contagion are "el mitín político, la reunión concejal o la discusión parlamentaria." The criticism Arguedas directs at these reunions approximates the kind of degeneracy theory critique he made of creole authors and their neurotic need to associate in groups, schools and movements.

The speech and neurological pathology diagnosed by Álvarez, Bunge and Arguedas is traced to both psychic and physiological origins. Particularly in the instances of Bunge and Arguedas this linkage has racial overtones as well. As enthusiastic ethnopsychologists, both were quick to attribute what they perceived as political chaos and corruption to the alleged psychological and biological faults of their national populations. [39] These faults were ascribed to the racially mixed *"gaucho"* or *"cholo"* of Argentina and Bolivia respectively. Following the degeneracy theories of Morel, Darwin and Le Bon regarding "hybrid" populations, Bunge and Arguedas posited that the mixed populations of Latin America were congenitally degenerate, and as such lacked the moral sense to distinguish between truth and fiction or the moral and the immoral. Thus, the argument goes, the mestizo-led governments of Latin America are physiologically and psychologically programmed for deception and simulation, and, concomitantly, the citizens ruled by these governments are congenitally conditioned to believe in their dissimulation.

This suspicion of a supposed racial inclination to perpetrating and believing in deception is deemed by Arguedas to be a central cause of national prostration:

> pero lo que de veras causa daños sin cuento, es la falta de probidad y honradez, porque los oradores no sólo se limitan ya a lucir el fuego de artificio de su elocuencia barata, sino que para imponerse, distinguirse y dominar, recurren al engaño, al fraude y a la mentira, porque adulan a las masas atribuyéndoles toda clase de atributos, cualidades y virtudes, halagando sus pasiones dominantes, fomentando sus vicios... (104)

In this passage from *Pueblo enfermo*, Arguedas' critique of corrupt bureaucrats and politicians rests upon racist and classist assumptions which he holds to be universal. Here Arguedas links political corruption or incompetence to the allegedly congenital faults he had previously assigned to what he perceives as the *cholo* bourgeois sector of Bolivian society. In this way, vices previously impugned to Bolivians of mixed ancestry, in this instance "verbomanía" and pathological lying, are simultaneously attributed to the emerging professional political class. That this class critique of

---

[39] Bunge states this rather succinctly in *Nuestra América* when he lists what he calls the "laws of life": *"Todas las manifestaciones de la vida de los pueblos son productos de psico-fisiología. Su psico-fisiología es de la herencia. La herencia lo es del medio natural. El medio natural obra en dos formas, ya directamente sobre el organismo estimulado por sus actividades, ya indirectamente, estimulándolas para la alimentación. Cuando estimula por sí al organismo, lo hace en un orden puramente fisio y psicológico; cuando lo estimula para la alimentación, en un orden doble, al propio tiempo fisio-psicológico y económico. Esto es todo"* (*sic* 160).

"labradores, mineros, abogadillos, propietarios, industriales, y pequeños capitalistas" is also implicitly associated with *cholo* psychological inadequacies, is verified by the immediately following para-
graph in which, as a partial solution to the problem, Arguedas proposes that the Bolivian government do all it can to foment European immigration.

At times Arguedas leaves his racial determinism to offer an insightful description of how the Bolivian elite maintains itself in
power to serve its own immediate interests. One such moment is
when Arguedas explains that one of the most important ways in
which a governmental representative maintains his power is to take
great pains to select people personally indebted to him to serve in
his jurisdiction, thus enabling undetected abuse of his office and
guaranteeing easy re-election. Yet such instances of analysis of the
social, political and material economy of corruption in Bolivia are
few and are interspersed among the overriding discourse of ethnic
pathology and simulation. It is out of this conviction that Arguedas
makes the following generalization: "En ese ambiente todo es simulación, prejuicio" (106). This is due, Arguedas argues, to the peculiar psychology of the Bolivian legislator:

> El diputado boliviano, insisto, surge de centros absolutamente
> nulos para la acción y no es el diestro conocedor de las necesi-
> dades del país; tampoco el estudioso erudito en la ciencia políti-
> ca y menos el agricultor o comerciante susceptible de hablar,
> pensar, discutir, y gobernar mediante las sanas advertencias de
> un sentido práctico, no; son abogadillos de vasta clientela mesti-
> za; empleados o parientes de empleados oficiales, escribidores
> vacuos y rimbombantes cuya sola habilidad consiste en halagar
> los instintos de las muchedumbres y atraerse por lo tanto, su
> simpatía. (106)

Here Arguedas mixes insightful commentary on the lack of a
national bourgeoisie or professional managerial class capable of
directing a modern, industrial national economy with racism. Although Arguedas sees it as a problem of education, he still clings
to pathological models of verbomania and degeneration through
association with "inferior" hybrid races, the "vasta clientela mestiza." Nevertheless Arguedas' analysis is also a critique of the ongoing feudal nature of Bolivian political institutions where family

ties are much more important than financial or technical knowledge. [40]

Arguedas characterizes the corrupt incompetence of the Bolivian legislature as a degenerate comedy or farce. He refers to the government as a "comic simulation" which conceals the weakness of the nation. The simulation itself is a danger to the nation, threatening the national body "de la cabeza a los pies." Significantly, Arguedas affirms that the pretense involved is not of a noble self-deluded quest for the ideal, as in the case of the laudable, aristocratic dementia of Don Quixote; rather he compares it to the mean-spirited, hypocritic, self-interested and decidedly middle class "perpetua mentira" of Molière's *Tartuffe*.

As with the case of the speech disorders of verbomania and onomatomania, the propensity for pathological behaviors of deception, usually ascribed to the individual, assume collective proportions in nations of alleged racial inferiority or, as Arguedas maintains: "El egoísmo individual, innato en esas razas, se acentúa colectivamente" (115). With this premise of national megalomania, Arguedas, in his conclusion to his chapter on governmental corruption, summarizes that a principal source of national illness is this will to deception and simulation, "ese particular estado de espíritu consistente en fingir un bienestar que no existe," resulting in a "simulación colectiva." Just as with the speech pathologies, this inclination to simulation is the product of a congenitally inferior, morally degenerate abulic personality. [41]

Another central target of Arguedas' attack against national enervation was the Bolivian press. In the chapter "La prensa, factor de

---

[40] In this sense Arguedas approximates, albeit for an entirely different ideological point of view, Agustín Cueva's analysis of the ongoing role of feudal oligarchies in Latin American nations which experienced the development of capitalism in limited "enclaves." In the following passage from *El desarrollo del capitalismo en América latina* Cueva states: "En aquellas sociedades en que el capitalismo se desarrolla en "enclaves," y en las que por lo tanto la supeditación del grueso del cuerpo social al capitalismo es meramente formal, los elementos feudales ocupan todavía el lugar que en las formaciones más avanzadas corresponde ya a los terratenientes de tipo "junker". Nos referimos naturalmente a países que mal que bien poseen un estado nacional, como Perú o Bolivia, y no a sociedades en las que el "enclave" se implanta mediante la ocupación extranjera" (133).

[41] Agustín Álvarez, in many instances Arguedas' predecessor, paraphrased the relationship between physiological and mental enervation and lying in his *Manual de patología política*: "El maximum de fraude y mentira coincide con el mínimum de energía física y viceversa..." (55).

corrupción colectiva," Arguedas diagrams the socially, morally and intellectually degrading role of the press in turn-of-the-century Bolivia. Arguedas' critique of the Bolivian press is particularly interesting because it involves elements of an auto-biographical self-defense against his detractors in the Bolivian press and sheds contemporary light on the history of Bolivian journalism and articulates a modern if not postmodern critique of the manipulation of signs, information and the formation of public opinion.

Arguedas' designation of the national press as a source of social corruption almost certainly contained an element of implicit autobiographical self-defense or what is colloquially referred to as "sour grapes." Beginning with the publication of his novel *Wata Wara* (1904), an account based on the historical Indian uprising of 1899, in part provoked by the brutal rape and murder of Wata Wara, a young Indian woman, at the hands of her landowner, Arguedas became the object of vehement criticism in the Bolivian press. The boldness of this novel is quite striking considering the state of national civil and race war convulsing Bolivia during the period. At this moment the liberal administration of Pando was engaged in a bloody war against the Aymyran democratic movement which sought the recognition of their lands and *ayllus* for which they held colonial titles (Albarracín Millán 93). The national press and influential intellectuals, such as Bautista Saavedra (also a future president of the republic), viewed the war as the final Spencerian conflict between the Indian and Bolivian nations (Albarracín Millán 94). To have written a novel based on this conflict, especially one in which the Indian uprising triumphs and results in the death of corrupt landowners, was an unforgivable offense to the anti-Indian creole and *mestizo* elite. The critical censure of the novel caused Arguedas considerable depression and on many occasions he sought to dismiss the novel as a "libro malo".[42]

Arguedas' adversarial relations with the national press were exacerbated by the publication of *Pueblo enfermo*. Without a doubt

---

[42] Albarracín Millán makes the argument that Arguedas' denunciations of *Wata Wara* may not have been sincere and that they might have constituted a strategy of provocation or a way of gaining renewed access to the public forum from which to launch new critiques. Albarracín Millán states: "El drama de arguedismo, espectacularmente contradictorio, tenía que pasar por estas pruebas positivamente desconcertantes para sus enemigos, pero gozosamente llevada adelante por el íntimo Arguedas que así veía realizarse su obra..." (95).

Arguedas provoked this attack by criticizing the press and the liberal government it supported as principal causes of national illness. [43] In *Pueblo enfermo* Arguedas states that anyone who points out the nation's problems is libeled as anti-patriotic. The press, Arguedas maintains, defines patriotism as continuing the great deception that all is well, that the nation is progressing: "El patriotismo consiste, ya se dijo, en mentir por lo grande, asegurando solemnemente y poniendo a los cielos por testigo, que el nivel moral sube incesantemente como caudal de río en otoño y marchan a maravilla sus instituciones..." (123). Those who break with this fiction are labeled as unpatriotic, and specifically in the case of Arguedas, a pessimist.

"Pessimist" is perhaps the most commonly employed epithet in discussions of Arguedas, or as one critic has stated: "Todo el mundo, el propio Arguedas incluído, está convencido que nuestro escritor fue un "pesimista"" (Roca 13). Thus Arguedas' vindication of the pessimist strongly suggests personal references. This is further evidenced by recurring allusions to the persecution of the pessimist in following chapters, with the word "pessimist" italicized, indicating an extra-textual referent as in this passage from the chapter "Causas de decadencia física": "Y quien diga lo contrario es un loco, un cándido, un *pesimista* (la palabra allí expresa mucho), y como tal, no hay que hacerle caso" (164). In summation, the sin of the pessimist is that he refuses to take part in the national propensity to lie or simulate.

Arguedas' distrust of the press, as well as his suspicion of political rhetoric, can be traced back to his readings of Le Bon. Le Bon undoubtedly reinforced Arguedas' belief that the problem of modern society was how to govern democratically in the presence of politically empowered masses whose main features are spontaneity and violence. In a society of accelerating secularization, Le Bon argued, the traditional and religious beliefs that governed society give way to new beliefs capable of structuring a society dominated by

---

[43] Ávila Echazú, in his *Resumen y antología de la literatura boliviana*, asserts that the role of the liberal press in Bolivia was to divert the attention of the population from substantive problems and to project the interests of the oligarchical mining elite as those of the nation: "Su papel director de la conciencia pública se encaminó a encubrir los intereses económicos antinacionales de la naciente oligarquía minera, a la cual le importaba muy poco la culturación de las masas" (86).

Obviously a similar criticism has been made of the role of the "free" press wherever capitalist liberal democracies prevail.

the "crowd." For this reason he stressed that it was very important to understand how the crowd conceived of itself and society, hence his *Psychology of the Crowd* (1895). In this work Le Bon argued that the masses think in a cloudy chain of interrelated images which have no relation to the original referent (Terán 19). This break between image and referent produces an effect of collective schizophrenia among the masses. Insofar as this mass schizophrenia is characterized by a space between the referent and the image, the crowd is more influenced by the imagery of communication than its content or, as Óscar Terán puts it, "En el espacio así abierto entre lo real y lo representado, lo que le impresiona según Le Bon a la imaginación popular 'no son los hechos en sí mismos, sino la manera en que son distribuídos'" (19).

Following from this argument, Arguedas' concern with deceptive or degenerate political rhetoric and sensationalist, misleading and sickly journalism, becomes clearer. Of the Bolivian press Arguedas states that it is "maleada en su base y no responde a sus primordiales fines eminentemente educadores" (117). In brief, Arguedas criticizes the Bolivian press for its superficial emphasis on information concerning such trivial activities as sports, cinema, and social events. The press is, Arguedas posits, responding to the interests of its new reading public. This new public's "mass psychology," according to Le Bon, inaugurates a new direction in press coverage in which the debased whims of the *nouveau riche* and the masses are flattered:

> Y gentes ayer de veras pobres, de veras malnacidas, cobran bríos con estas marcas de adulación de otras gentes bajas; y sus periódicos, agresivos de escándalo, reflejan entonces sus almas ordinarias porque emplean el insulto soez, la insinuación perversa, el gracejo fácil del arroyo, gastan chistes vulgares, se muestran insolentes, agresivos y acometedores para quien desdeña tomarlos en cuenta y no responde nunca a sus ataques de trastienda sucia, así como se les ve sumisos, serviles, ruines y bajos para el fuerte que manda o maneja un negocio y puede pagarles dinero para acallar sus campañas... (121)

If the sexually degenerate overtones of this diatribe against the press and its prurient readership was not obvious to the reader of *Pueblo enfermo*, witness the references to things "low," "crude," "perverse," "vulgar," "dirty," and "base," then Arguedas made this allusion to sexual enervation strikingly clear in an assertion that leaves no room for doubt: "Su lectura es, por eso, embrutecedora, como la masturbación" (130). Like the contemporary medical warnings against masturbation, the vice of the press is addictive. It causes a "fascinación maníaca" which "degenera hasta manía" (131) in small towns. In the light of this discourse of degenerative masturbation one can only wonder at the intention of the following affirmation: "yo coloco a la prensa como uno de los órganos más activos de la disolución moral de un pueblo..." (140). Like the organs of those who compulsively masturbate against medical injunctions, the press is the most "active organ" of national degeneration.

Only at the end of the chapter on the morally corrupting influence of Bolivian journalism does Arguedas touch upon, albeit briefly, the concrete historical and political damage caused by this addictive, degenerate misinformation. As a vice, the press is seductive and therefore it is believed without question. To further substantiate this point Arguedas quotes from a speech by the Scottish historian Thomas Macaulay who was very critical of the role of the press in the parliamentary system. Arguedas maintains that the role of the press is similarly injurious to the Bolivian political system. Inasmuch as Arguedas considers the majority of the reading public to be morally, psychologically and congenitally inferior, he posits that they are prone to the mania of believing whatever they read. This holds true, he asserts, for "el pueblo, burgueses y hasta capitalistas." Arguedas briefly states, in this 1937 edition of *Pueblo enfermo*, that the cost of this vice has been the destructive Chaco war with Paraguay. For Arguedas the seductive vice of degenerate simulation and national megalomania in the press is, in large measure, responsible for this national debacle:

> esta guerra fatal para Bolivia y que en ningún caso podría ser provechosa para el país, ha sido alentada por toda la prensa, sin excepción, y que la prensa, unida a la obcecación, ceguera e incomprensión de ese mismo Salamanca y de los técnicos militares, ha producido el espantoso desastre que hoy contemplamos... y lamentamos. (144)

Another principal source of debilitating simulation addressed in *Pueblo enfermo* is ostentation or "el boato." This alleged psychological need for ostentation is linked into Arguedas' larger premise of national megalomania; if Bolivians have delusions of grandeur, the argument goes, then they must manifest it in exhibitions of wealth and luxury. Following Bunge, whom he credits with the discovery, Arguedas alleges that the inclination for ostentation is an inherent feature of mestizo psychology. This tendency, Arguedas argues, is due in part to the inheritance of Iberian arrogance, as detailed by Bunge in *Nuestra América*, as well as to the mestizo's desire for social legitimization and advancement.

Through a form of anthropological analysis, Bunge and Arguedas avow that ostentation is an instrument of power for the mestizo population. For both of these authors, a conspicuous and ornamental display of power is an indication of inferiority or uncertainty. Arguedas describes how morally and intellectually bankrupt bureaucrats, legislators and military officials are compelled to "*hacerse retratar* con todas las insignias de su cargo" (*sic* 226). This vanity is itself classified by Arguedas as "aparentismo" and "aparentamiento," conditions in which governmental officials who are "desprovistos de méritos personales" assume their position through lavish dress, arrogant behavior and luxurious living. Arguedas infers that this is an archetypal, nearly universal feature of inferior individuals who, unlike the truly gifted individuals who earn their position through silent, humble and diligent labor, must dress themselves up in power in a form of megalomaniacal transvestism. Arguedas reports that changing times have made the courtly ostentation of the past impossible for twentieth century *caudillos* who must compensate for this loss with formally posed studio photographs.

Despite the moral and racial nonsense of Arguedas' analysis, his credible account of the changing codes of official ostentation suggests another, non-racial or non-psychological explanation. In effect, what we observe in this account is the conflictive transformation of a socio-historical sensibility concerning the legitimization and expression of power. Specifically, we witness the shift from the vestiges of colonial, feudal and viceregal authority, one which constantly makes use of pomp and ceremony to both legitimize and enact its power, to the mythology of the rule of the naturally meritorious within liberal democracy whose power is based on supposed claims of innate superiority of intelligence and morality, thus requiring fewer, or at least different, ceremonial proofs.

Arguedas traces the origin of ostentation in political life to the lavish dressing of mestiza women in their attempt to mimic and break into relatively white or *castizo*, elite, feminine social circles. According to Arguedas, these traditional, feminine, oligarchical circles maintained considerable socio-cultural or symbolic power and continued to exclude mestiza women despite the fact that mixed race *caudillos* held political power. In fact Arguedas declares that one such *caudillo*, Belzú, inaugurated a civil war out of resentment of his exclusion from such genteel societies. The very continuity of such civil conflicts, Arguedas posits, along with the "lower" and "vulgar" people they bring to power, makes it difficult for the *caudillo du jour* and his entourage to distinguish themselves from the "mob" in the absence of the former's racial superiority. In this vacuum of political semiotics Arguedas singles out the *mestiza* who vainly tries to mimic or simulate the "graciousness" of feminine elite symbolic capital through an interpretation of crass ostentation, but who in reality recreates the value system of the "lowly" Indian:

> Y entonces el elemento femenil de esos grupos de flamante formación, recurrió a la riqueza del boato como medio de adquirir prestigio e imponerse a las masas y aun a los mismos círculos dominadores, imitando así a las clases indígenas, para las que un miembro tiene más valor cuanto mayor sea el precio de su traje, esto es, y como lo dice bellamente el generoso don Quijote: "que está la diferencia, en que unos fueron, ya que no son, y otros son, que ya no fueron." (149)

THE DISCOURSE OF "PUBLIC HEALTH" IN *PUEBLO ENFERMO*: ITS RACIAL, MORAL AND CLASS UNDERPINNINGS

It is easy for the present day reader of *Pueblo enfermo* to dismiss it as the work of a racist crank and polemicist who promoted scientifically invalid, anti-social and morally repugnant theories about the ethnic composition of Bolivia and Latin America. Surely, the modern critic thinks, such theories have long been disproved and only present day extremists and irrational racists would embrace such nonsense. [44] Obviously there is a great deal of truth in this

---

[44] Martin Stabb, in his overview of *Pueblo enfermo,* gives the impression that views such as those expressed by Arguedas no longer enjoy scientific credibility. In

comforting opinion. Nevertheless, to regard the theories of racial degeneration as anachronistic misses the point that in some instances these theories have merely been transformed in keeping with ongoing developments in the discourses of social science and medicine.

Specifically, I am referring to what can be called the discourse of "Public Health" in *Pueblo enfermo*. Apart from the blatant arguments based on discredited theories of race and geographical determinism, Arguedas employs the allied discourses of social reform and public health to address what he perceived as the interrelated problems of crime, madness, alcoholism, malnutrition, fertility, venereal disease, bodily hygiene and public sanitation. The concepts and methodologies Arguedas employed to address these issues, namely notions of congenital inclination, pathological cause and effect, and statistical analysis, are still very much in use today.

The damaging effects of vice were very much a concern for Arguedas. Yet just whether it was a case of vices debilitating the individual, or the case of already degenerate individuals and races manifesting their inferiority through an inclination for vice, is unclear. Medical and psychological science resolved this ambiguity with the invention of new illnesses which accounted for these vices. Examples of such nineteenth-century creations are dipsomania for drunkenness, and kleptomania and pyromania for criminal activity (Carlson 130). In all of these conditions an alleged innate lack of morality manifests itself in pathologies of the will. Not coincidentally, this was the same soul-less lack of morality impugned to women, the working class and the so-called inferior races by nineteenth-century degeneracy theory. This congenital deficiency was believed to make these groups vulnerable to the vices or illnesses of promiscuous sex, liquor and crime (Nye 60). In this sense degeneracy theory led social critics such as Arguedas to find the source of the nation's social and economic problems in the medically constructed figures of the alcoholic, the criminal, the prostitute, the syphilitic degenerate and the unhygienic worker.

---

his book *In Quest of Identity. Patterns in the Spanish American Essay of Ideas. 1890-1960* Stabb affirms: "As we shall see, much of the theorizing which found in miscegenation the *causa causarum* of the continent's ills was of relatively short duration; few writers of recent decades have held to racistic interpretations of Spanish American reality" (23).

In his chapter on indigenous psychology, and even more so in the chapter "Causas de decadencia física," Arguedas points to alcoholism and the alcoholic as central causes of national illness. In regard to the indigenous population, Arguedas states that they are prone to alcoholism as the result of their prior, historically acquired degenerate state: "Exasperada la raza indígena, abatida, gastada física y moralmente, inhábil para intentar la violenta reivindicación de sus derechos, hase entregado al alcoholismo de manera alarmante" (51). Provided the voluminous historical record documenting the real problem that aboriginal peoples have had with Western liquor, it is difficult to deconstruct Arguedas' sympathetic, purely psychological explanation. However, the interesting footnote to this quote helps us to understand the social needs and sensibility behind the historical construction of "the alcoholic."

In this long footnote based on an article by Miguel de Unamuno, Arguedas suggests that alcoholism among the Indians is traceable to their slower pace of evolution which has not kept up with either European progress or vice. But the really interesting assertion in this passage on alcoholism does not deal with its etiology, but rather with alcoholism's incompatibility with the requirements of modern industrial life. In an article published in *La Nación*, which is quoted at length in *Pueblo enfermo* Unamuno states, or rather suggests for our further interpretation, that the problem with alcoholism and the reason for its historical construction as a social problem and medical disease is that it constitutes an obstacle to the increased demands for social discipline in the modern industrial workplace; Unamuno states: "La vida de civilización, con su complejidad creciente, con la multitud de acomodaciones sensoriales y volitivas que exige, pide un sistema nervioso de una cierta complejidad también" (52).

Arguedas backs up this assertion by providing what can be described as a *costumbrismo* of alcoholism in Bolivia. He enters into detail explaining the customs of Bolivian bar, or "cantina" culture and the cultural requirements that insist upon the obligatory serving and consumption of liquor at all social occasions and meetings including even the most casual social visits. Such indulgence, Arguedas maintains, breeds counter-productive sloth in what should be the most disciplined of social classes, the bourgeoisie: "La holgazanería es un vicio harto común, especialmente en la clase media de la sociedad" (167). Just like their fellow class members who profit from the trade in liquor the middle-class alcoholic is dragged down by his supposed congenital, *mestizo* inclination to drink, or as Arguedas states he "cede a las llamadas de sus instintos salvajes y a las exigencias de sus gustos atávicos" (167).

As for the Indian peasants, Arguedas associates their alleged state of immoral, unproductive inebriation with the promiscuous orgies of irrationality suggestive of traditional, pre-industrial rites of carnival. Yet underlying this moral and social critique of non-pro-ductivity one discerns another more contemporary political con-cern. Specifically, Arguedas' dislike of these syncretic "fiestas indí-genas" is undoubtedly linked to their role in the maintenance of so-cial, political, economic and cultural relations among the various in-digenous communities. In this function, the fiesta calendar also served as a catalyst for military mobilization during the many Indi-an uprisings of the late nineteenth century (Platt 319). Reproducing at length a passage from a study by the historian José Manuel Cortés, a work that Arguedas admits was already seventy-five years out of date, Arguedas partakes of the kind of classist, moral outrage at popular gatherings typical of the discourse of public health at the turn-of-the-century; Cortés states:

> La plebe de Cochabamba vive casi en perpetua orgía y tiene, por consiguiente, todos los vicios, todo el descaro que la em-briaguez trae consigo. Del lunes, en que continúa la borrachera del domingo, se ha hecho un santo, con el nombre de San Lunes: este santo de la beodez está pintado encima de las puer-tas de las chicherías; la cara es de un ebrio; un cántaro de chicha forma el cuerpo; un violín y una guitarra, los brazos; no tiene pies, sin duda para denotar la dificultad con que caminan los borrachos ... (169)

In keeping with this discourse of social discipline and morality, Arguedas finds that one positive development for the battle against degenerative alcoholism in Bolivia is the emergence of sports in the national landscape. Here physical exercise and fresh air assume the nationally therapeutic functions of literally "airing-out" the conse-quences of old bad habits and of instilling the structures of physical and mental discipline necessary to engage in both sports and the modern workplace, an assertion Arguedas makes explicit in the fol-lowing passage: "...y es el deporte el que va matando al vicio y creando hábitos de disciplina, noción de responsabilidad, deberes de ayuda mutua y de solidaridad" (170).

For Arguedas, the disciplining and modernization of the Bolivian population also meant subjecting it to the new social codes for personal and public hygiene. In his desire to stamp out filth and vice Arguedas expresses the same kind of frustrations voiced by medically-minded reformers in Europe. This is particularly true in the case of individual bodily hygiene or bathing. Needless to say, in his discussion on the customs of national hygiene Arguedas does not consider the impact of a lack of a universal and dependable water supply, indoor plumbing or such banal items as soap. His argument is, as always purely psychological. Nevertheless his complaints that the lower classes resisted bathing on superstitious grounds and out of previously established scientific injunctions against total immersion in water echo the experiences of social reformers in France.[45]

Arguedas' complaint about the unhealthy filth piled up in Bolivia's capital of La Paz could have been written by social reformers of the same period about any major cosmopolitan center in the world, particularly in those metropolises of the periphery where municipal poverty and a lack of orchestrated sanitation combined to make for unhealthy living conditions as described in the following passage from *Pueblo enfermo*: "Tirando por cualquier lado de la ciudad, a poco andar, se tropieza con muladares repulsivos donde se pudren, al aire libre, cadáveres de perros, asnos y caballos" (173).

Arguedas does not differentiate between literal filth and vice as he attributes the increase in mortality rates to alcoholism and unhygienic conditions. In this case, the scientific and historical veracity of Arguedas' assertion is not in doubt, nor are his sound remarks about problems in nutrition the mere products of a discursive shift or changing perception. This credibility only underlines the fact

---

[45] As Alain Corbin notes in *The Foul and the Fragrant. Odor and the French Social Imagination*, the importance of the psychological resistance to hygiene cannot be underestimated: "The relative indifference shown by the French to cleanliness, their rejection of water, their long tolerance of strong bodily odors, and their continued privatization of excrement and rubbish cannot be explained solely by a secret distrust of innovation, by relative poverty, or by slow urbanization. It was a collective attitude towards the body, the organic functions, and the sensory messages that governed behavior patterns" (173).

that we are still within the conceptual framework of public health articulated by Arguedas and are sometimes blind to its more class-based and racist criticisms of the masses. This is a framework which explains social, economic problems in terms of morality and pathology and national problems in terms of sick individuals who are dragging the nation down.

Reviewing what he classifies as the causes of national decadence and the origin of the nation's "modo de pensar tan primitivo, tan sin substancia, tan *enfermo*" [sic]: alcoholism, the lack of hygiene, malnutrition and venereal disease, Arguedas states the premise of his public health discourse: "pues los fenómenos sociales hay que explicarlos biológicamente..." (175). This assertion that the circumstantially acquired "vices" or "illnesses" of prostitution, crime and alcoholism can be passed on to future generations is premised upon a Lamarckian concept of evolution. Moreover, the results of this transmission, following Morel's theory of progressivity, are that the effects of such inherited vices become more acute with each generation (Carlson 122).

For Arguedas the consequences of this process are quite damning for Bolivia's national health and lead him to make the following pessimistic diagnosis and prognosis:

> ...debemos convenir franca, corajudamente, sin ambages, que estamos *enfermos*, o mejor que hemos nacido enfermos y que nuestra disolución pueda ser cierta, no como pueblo, porque esto, sin ser imposible, sería difícil, sino como raza, o más bien, como conjunto de individuos con unos mismos anhelos e idéntica conformación mental. (*sic* 176)

In a surprisingly indifferent follow-up to this conclusion, one which Arguedas expresses "sin pasión y fríamente," he concludes that this is how evolution works. The one thing which could save Bolivia, a remedy which he claims has saved several other Latin American nations, would be a massive wave of European immigration which could serve as a catalyst for the growth of industry, agriculture and commerce. But, as always with Arguedas, the basis of this cure is racial.

CONCLUSION

Thus there are innumerable healths of the body; and the more
we allow the unique and incomparable to raise its head again,
and the more we abjure the dogma of the "equality of men," the
more must the concept of a *normal* health, along with a normal
diet and the normal course of an illness, be abandoned by medical men. Only then would the time have come to reflect on the
health and illness of the *soul*, and to find the peculiar virtue of
each man in the health of his soul. (*The Gay Science* 177)

Nietzsche's admonition that there are "innumerable healths of
the body," strikes me as an appropriate note with which to conclude my consideration of the discourse of national illness in turn-
of-the-century Spain and Latin America. The cultural, ethnic, and
regional diversity invoked by such a broad discursive field necessarily transcends the imposition of a universal doctrine of cultural
health. Indeed, the three texts which have constituted the principal
basis of this study, the Spaniard Ángel Ganivet's *Idearium español*,
the Uruguayan José Enrique Rodó's *Ariel*, and the Bolivian Alcides
Arguedas' *Pueblo enfermo*, came out of specific national configurations which resist generalization. The polarities of health and illness
which these texts addressed corresponded to the particular divi-
sions of ethnicity, gender and class found in these nations. Within
the discourse of national illness, these differences were perceived as
threats to political unity, economic growth and cultural autonomy.
Thus the abstract and indirect allusions to regional difference in the
Spain of Ganivet's *Idearium español*, euphemistically attributed to
the vagaries of a geographical spirit, contrast sharply with the cen-

trality given to a detailed science of racial hybridity in the Bolivia of Arguedas' *Pueblo enfermo*.

Somewhere between these two lies Rodó's *Ariel*, a seemingly idealized treatment of Latin American regeneration which rested heavily on the theories of degeneracy inscribed in the polarized figures of Caliban and Ariel. As I have argued, despite Rodó's substantial redirection of the onus of this degeneracy, his underlying reliance on organicist conceptions of health and his flight from the body and the calibanesque masses situates him within the discourse of national illness. In this light it is important to reiterate that the focus of this study has been on the psychological, medical and evolutionary terminology of degeneration, and not merely on its political intent.

Among the many theories of racial, psychological, philosophical and physiological enervation deployed in these texts, the underlying and unifying concept of these discourses of illness was that they stemmed from pathologies of the will. Across the intellectual disciplines, issues of alleged racial inferiority, sexual debilitation and evolutionary progress were premised on the healthy exercise of volitional energy. Throughout the consideration of these texts we have seen how the vital functioning of the will has been linked to race, gender, immaturity and heredity. Significantly, we have also observed that these categories have not been conceptualized in isolation from one another, but rather they have operated in a complementary manner.

Thus, as I have argued, the pathology of the will Arguedas impugned to indigenous and mestizo Americans in *Pueblo enfermo* was primarily racial. However, the scientific articulation of this notion was based on characterological assumptions concerning the youth, virility and environment of these groups in turn-of-the-century Bolivia. The crucial issue for thinkers such as Arguedas, Rodó and Ganivet was to determine whether these perceived infirmities of the will were essential or circumstantial. For Arguedas there was little doubt that Bolivia was condemned by its racial composition.

Rodó, as evidenced in *Ariel*, also conceived of national health in terms of the health of the will. Yet while Arguedas believed the perceived racial immaturity of Bolivia to be an essential impediment to volitional health, Rodó conceived of Latin America's youth as a developmental stage full of vitality and promise. Working with the same theoretical tools of degeneracy theory as did Arguedas, Rodó arrived at different conclusions. For Rodó, the healthy exercise of the will required the proper cultivation of youth in a masculine setting away from women and the masses. In the heady, homoerotic and anxious classroom setting of *Ariel*, Prospero, the mentor of youth, tells his students that cultural regeneration, following the ideas of Schopenhauer, Fouillée and others, departs from the volitional act of believing in the power of their youth. The tension within Rodó's championing of youth as a source of healing energy comes from the concomitant association of the will, particularly during puberty, with sexual awakening. Thus in *Ariel* the strength of the will and its ability to transform the social body is linked to youth in potentially positive terms, provided that this "tesoro" is chastely guarded.

This last point leads us back to Ganivet and the linkage between the Spanish and Latin American discourses of national illness. As mentioned during my discussion of *Idearium español*, Ganivet also considered Latin America to be in a developmental stage of youth. For Ganivet, the youth of Latin America was intimately tied to the "virginity" of Spain. In this sense, Ganivet's defense of Spain was far from disinterested inasmuch as he conceived of Latin America as a youthful component of a superficially senile, yet spiritually young or pure, Hispanic character. In Latin America Ganivet found hope for the spiritual regeneration of Spain, referring to the latter as "la promesa de una futura superioridad de nuestra raza."

The shared conceptual preconditions for the linkage between Latin American youth and Spanish virginity was the promotion of chastity and the conservation of what Fouillée had termed "vital internal energy." The failure to conserve this energy led to listlessness and a lack of volitional energy, what Ganivet diagnosed as aboulia. While this connection of chastity retained the specificity of the long colonial relationship between Spain and the Americas, the linkage between unsanctioned or excessive sexual activity and pathologies of the will was a commonly held belief in turn-of-the-century degeneracy theory.

This connection between Spain and Latin America also gave greater impetus to a reconsideration of the character faults attributed to Spanish and Latin American peoples by the Black Legend. This old slander of the Spanish character was reactivated in the discursive field by turn-of-the-century notions of heredity which posited that the sins of the Spanish conquistadors were genetically transmitted to Latin Americans. In the political sphere this idea was resuscitated by the rhetoric of racial character surrounding the Spanish-American War of 1898. The congenital faults of an alleged, underlying, transatlantic Hispanic character and the discourse of racial inferiority generated by the disaster of '98, interpellated Spaniards and Latin Americans alike in a shared discourse of characterological degeneration. As I have argued, it is not a shared ideological response to this interpellation which brings the three diverse authors I have examined together, but rather the compulsion to respond within the terminology of this interpellation, namely the discourse of national illness. I close this study with this chestnut from Nordau, that staunch and unintentionally amusing figure of discourse of degeneration: "Our long and sorrowful wandering through the hospital – for as such we have recognised, if not all civilized humanity, at all events the upper stratum of the population of large towns to be – is ended" (536).

BIBLIOGRAPHY

Achugar, Hugo. *Poesía y Sociedad.* Montevideo: Arca, 1985.

Adorno, Theodor W. *Prisms.* Trans. Samuel and Shierry Weber. Cambridge: MIT Press, 1982.

Albarracín Millán, Juan. *Alcides Arguedas: la conciencia crítica de una época.* La Paz: Ediciones Réplica, 1979.

Altamira, Rafael de. *Psicología del pueblo español.* Barcelona: Editorial Minerva, 1917 edition.

Althusser, Louis. "Idéologie et Appareils Idéologiques d'Etat." *La Pensée* 151 (1970): 3-38.

Álvarez, Agustín. *Manual de patología política.* Buenos Aires: La Cultura Argentina, 1916.

Anderson, Robert K. "El simbolismo universal en *Ariel.*" *Hispanic Journal,* vol. 12, no. 1 (Spring 1991): 87-95.

Arguedas, Alcides. *Pueblo enfermo.* Santiago: Ediciones Ercilla, 1937.

Ávila Echazú, Edgar. *Resumen y antología de la literatura boliviana.* La Paz: Editores Gisbert & Cía, 1973.

Benedetti, Mario. *Genio y figura de José Enrique Rodó.* Buenos Aires: Editorial Universitaria de Buenos Aires, 1966.

Beverley, John. *Del Lazarillo al Sandinismo: Estudios sobre la función ideológica de la literatura española e hispanoamericana.* Minneapolis: Institute for the Study of Ideologies and Literature/Prisma Institute, 1987.

——— and Zimmerman, Marc. *Literature and Politics in the Central American Revolutions.* Austin: University of Texas Press, 1990.

Brotherston, Gordon. Introduction. *Ariel.* By José Enrique Rodó. Cambridge: Cambridge University Press, 1967.

Bunge, Carlos Octavio. *Nuestra América.* Buenos Aires: Casa Vaccaro, 1918.

Busst, A.F.L. "The Image of the Androgyne in the Nineteenth Century." *Romantic Mythologies.* Ed. Ian Fletcher. New York: Barnes and Noble, 1967. 1-95.

Carlson, Eric T. "Medicine and Degeneration: Theory and Praxis." *Degeneration: The Dark Side of Progress.* Eds. J. Edward Chamberlin and Sander L. Gilman. New York: Columbia University Press, 1985.

Casalla, Mario. *América en el pensamiento de Hegel. Admiración y rechazo.* Buenos Aires: Catálogos, 1992.

de Certau, Michel. *The Writing of History.* Trans. Tim Conley. New York: Columbia University Press, 1988.

Concha, Jaime. "El *Ariel* de Rodó, O Juventud, 'Humano Tesoro'." *Nuevo Texto Crítico,* vol. V, nos. 9/10 (1992): 121-134.

Corbin, Alain. *The Foul and the Fragrant. Odor and the French Social Imagination.* NY: Berg Publishers Ltd, 1986.

Costa Lima, Luiz. "A Ficção Oblíqua: *The Tempest.*" *Nuevo Texto Crítico,* vol. V, nos. 9/10 (1992): 85-102.

Crawford, William Rex. *A Century of Latin American Thought.* Cambridge: Harvard UP, 1967.

Cueva, Agustín. *El desarrollo del capitalismo en América latina.* Mexico: Siglo XXI, 1985 edition.

Curtius, Ernst Robert. *European Literature and the Latin Middle Ages.* Trans. Williard R. Trask. Princeton: Princeton University Press, 1973.

Darío, Rubén. "Max Nordau." *Rubén Darío. Obras Completas,* vol. 2. Madrid: Afrodisio Aguado, 1950-53.

Dellamora, Richard. *Masculine Desire. The Sexual Politics of Victorian Aestheticism.* Chapel Hill: The University of North Carolina Press, 1990.

Díaz Arguedas, Julio. *Alcides Arguedas, el incomprendido.* La Paz: Ediciones Isla, 1978.

Díaz-Plaja, Guillermo. *Modernismo frente a noventa y ocho. Una introducción a la literatura española del siglo XX.* Madrid: Espasa-Calpe, S.A., 1966.

Dijkstra, Bram. *Idols of Perversity. Fantasies of Feminine Evil in Fin-De-Siecle Culture.* New York: Oxford University Press, 1986.

Durán Luzio, Juan. *Creación y Utopía. Letras de Hispanoamérica.* Costa Rica: Editorial de la Universidad Nacional, 1979.

Dussel, Enrique. "Eurocentrism and Modernity (Introduction to the Frankfurt Lectures)." *The Postmodernism Debate in Latin America.* Eds. John Beverley, José Oviedo and Michael Aronna. Durham: Duke University Press, 1995.

Earle, Peter G. and Mead, Robert Jr. *Historia del Ensayo Latinoamericano.* Mexico: Ediciones de Andrea, 1973.

Felski, Rita. "The Counterdiscourse of the Feminine in Three Texts by Wilde, Huysmans and Sacher-Masoch." *PMLA,* vol. 106, no. 5 (1991): 1094-1105.

Fernández, Teodosio. *Los géneros ensayísticos hispanoamericanos.* Madrid: Taurus, 1990.

Fernández Retamar, Roberto. *Calibán. Apuntes sobre la cultura en nuestra América.* Mexico: Editorial Diógenes, S.A., 1972.

Foucault, Michel. *The Birth of the Clinic. An Archaeology of Medical Perception.* Trans. A.M. Sheridan Smith. New York: Vintage Books, 1975.

———. *The History of Sexuality. Volume I: An Introduction.* Trans. Robert Hurley. New York: Vintage Books, 1978.

Fouillée, Alfred. *La Psychologie des Idées-Forces.* 2 vols. Paris: F. Alcan, 1893.

Fox, E. Inman. Introducción. *Idearium español.* By Ángel Ganivet. Madrid: Colección Austral, 1990. 9-39.

Franco, Jean. *The Modern Culture of Latin America: Society and the Artist.* Harmondsworth: Penguin, 1970.

Francovich, Guillermo. *Alcides Arguedas y otros ensayos sobre la historia.* La Paz: Librería Editorial "Juventud," 1979.

Freud, Sigmund. *Civilization and its Discontents.* Trans. James Strachey. New York: W.W. Norton & Company, Inc., 1961.

Ganivet, Ángel. *Idearium español.* Madrid: Colección Austral, 1990 ed.

———. *Granada la Bella.* Granada: Editorial Don Quijote, 1981.

———. *Obras Completas.* Ed. Melchor Fernández Almagro. 2 vols. Madrid: Aguilar, 1943; 2nd ed., 1959; 3rd ed., 1961.

García-Nieto, María Carmen. *La crisis del sistema canovista, 1898-1923.* Madrid: Guadiana, 1972.

García-Nieto, María Carmen. *Restauración y desastre, 1874-1898.* Madrid: Guadiana, 1972.

Gerbi, Antonello. *The Dispute of America.* Trans. Jeremy Moyle. Pittsburgh: University of Pittsburgh Press, 1973.

Gilman, Sander L. *Pathology and Difference* Ithaca: Cornell University Press, 1985.

———. "Sexology, Psychoanalysis, and Degeneration: From a Theory of Race to a Race Theory." *Degeneration: The Dark Side of Progress.* Eds. J. Edward Chamberlin and Sander L. Gilman. New York: Columbia University Press, 1985.

Gilman, Stuart C. "Political Theory and Degeneration: From Left to Right, From Up to Down." *Degeneration: The Dark Side of Progress.* Eds. J. Edward Chamberlin and Sander L. Gilman. New York: Columbia University Press, 1985.

Ginsberg, Judith. *Angel Ganivet.* London: Tamesis, 1985.

González Echevarría, Roberto. *The Voice of the Masters: Writing and Authority in Modern Latin America.* Austin: University of Austin, 1985.

Gutiérrez Girardot, Rafael. *Modernismo.* Barcelona: Montesinos, 1983.

Harding, F.J.W. *Jean-Marie Guyau (1854-1888). Aesthetician and Sociologist. A Study of his Aesthetic Theory and Critical Practice.* Geneva: Librairie Droz, 1973.

Harris, Olivia. "Ethnic Identity and Market Relations: Indians and Mestizos in the Andes." *Ethnicity, Markets, and Migration in the Andes. At the Crossroads of History and Anthropology.* Eds. Brooke Larson and Olivia Harris, Durham: Duke University Press, 1995.

Hathorn, Richmond. *Classical Mythology.* Beirut: The American University of Beirut, 1977.

Hegel. *Lectures on the Philosophy of World History.* Trans. H.B. Nisbet. Cambridge: Cambridge University Press, 1975.

———. "Philosophy of Nature." *Hegel: The Essential Writings.* Ed. Frederick G. Weiss. New York: Harper Torchbooks, 1974.

Henríquez Ureña, Pedro. "La cultura de las humanidades." *La utopía de América.* Caracas: Biblioteca Ayacucho, 1978.

Herrero, Javier. "Spain as Virgin: Radical Traditionalism in Angel Ganivet." *Homenaje a Juan López-Morillas.* Eds. José Amor y Vázquez and A. David Kossoff. Madrid: Gredos, 1982. 247-256.

Huysmans, Joris-Karl. *Against Nature.* Trans. Robert Baldick. London: Penguin Books, 1959.

Janaway, Chistopher. *Self and World in Schopenhauer's Philosophy.* New York: Oxford University Press, 1989.

Jenkyns, Richard. *The Victorians and Ancient Greece.* Cambridge: Harvard University Press, 1980.

Jitrik, Noe. *Las contradicciones del modernismo.* Mexico: El Colegio de México, 1978.

Jurkevich, Gayana. "*Abulia,* Nineteenth-Century Psychology and the Generation of 1898." *Hispanic Review,* vol. 60, no. 2 (Spring 1992): 181-194.

Kant. *Observations on the Feeling of the Beautiful and Sublime.* Trans. John T. Goldthwait. Berkeley: University of California Press, 1965.

Krafft-Ebing, Richard von. *Psychopathia Sexualis.* Brooklyn: Physicians and Surgeons Book Co., 1926.

Labanyi, Jo. "Nation, Narration, Naturalization: A Barthesian Critique of the 1898 Generation." *New Hispanisms: Literature, Culture, Theory.* Eds. Mark Millington and Paul Julian Smith. Ottawa: Dovehouse Editions, 1995.

Lastra, Pedro. "Las contradicciones de Alcides Arguedas," in *Relecturas Hispanoamericanas.* Chile: Editorial Universitaria, 1987. 51-62.

Lazo, Raimundo. "Estudio Preliminar," in *Ariel. Liberalismo y Jacobinismo.* By José Enrique Rodó. Mexico: Editorial Porrúa, 1977.

Le Bon, Gustave. *The Crowd; A Study of the Popular Mind*. London: E. Benn Ltd., 1930.

————. *Gustave Le Bon, the man and his works: a presentation with introduction, first translations into English, and edited extracts by Alice Walker*. Indianapolis: Liberty Press, 1978.

————. *The Psychology of Peoples*. New York: Stechert, 1924.

Litvak, Lily. *A Dream of Arcadia: Anti-Industrialism in Spanish Literature*. Austin and London: University of Texas Press, 1975.

Lombroso, Cesare and Ferrero, William. *The Female Offender*. London: T. Fisher, 1895.

Lukács, G. "On the Nature and Form of the Essay." *Soul and Form*. Cambridge: MIT Press, 1974.

Marichal, Juan. *Cuatro fases de la historia intelectual latinoamericana*. Madrid: Ediciones Cátedra, 1978.

Martí, José. "Nuestra América." *Política de Nuestra América*. Mexico: Siglo Veintiuno, 1989. 37-52.

Martínez Cuadrado, Miguel. *La burguesía conservadora (1874-1931)*. Madrid: Alianza Editorial/Alfaguara, 1986.

Melis, Antonio. "Entre Ariel y Calibán, ¿Próspero?" *Nuevo Texto Crítico*, vol. V, nos. 9/10 (1992): 113-119.

Molloy, Sylvia. "Too Wilde for Comfort: Desire and Ideology in Fin-de-Siecle Spanish America." *Social Text*, nos. 31/32, 1992.

Montero, Óscar. "Translating Decadence: Julián del Casal's Reading of Huysmans and Moreau." *Revista de Estudios Hispánicos* 26 (1992): 369-389.

Montes Huidobro, Matías. "El dogma de la Inmaculada Concepción como interpretación de la mujer en la obra de Ganivet." *Duquesne Hispanic Review* 13 (1968): 9-25.

Mosse, George L. *Nationalism and Sexuality. Middle Class Morality and Sexual Norms in Modern Europe*. New York: Howard Fertig, 1985.

Nietzsche. *The Birth of Tragedy and the Case of Wagner*. Trans. Walter Kaufman. New York: Vintage Books, 1967.

————. *The Gay Science*. Trans. Walter Kaufman. New York: Vintage Books, 1974.

————. *On the Genealogy of Morals*. Trans. Walter Kaufman. New York: Vintage Books, 1969.

Nixon, Rob. "Caribbean and African Appropriations of *The Tempest*." *Critical Inquiry* 13 (Spring 1987): 557-578.

Nordau, Max. *Degeneration*. New York: Appleton, 1895.

Nye, Robert A. "Sociology and Degeneration: The Irony of Progress." *Degeneration: The Dark Side of Progress*, Eds. J. Edward Chamberlin and Sander L. Gilman. New York: Columbia University Press, 1985.

Ochoa Antich, Nancy. *La mujer en el pensamiento liberal*. Quito: Editorial El Conejo, 1987.

Olmedo Moreno, Miguel. *El pensamiento de Ganivet*. Madrid: Revista de Occidente, 1965.

Orringer, Nelson. "Towards a Theory of the Body: Ortega and His Sources." *Ortega y Gasset and the Question of Modernity*. Ed. Patrick H. Dust. Minneapolis: The Prisma Institute, 1989. 127-151.

Ortiz, Fernando. *Los negros brujos. Apuntes para un estudio de etnología criminal*. Madrid: Editorial-América, 1917.

Pedreira, Antonio. *Insularismo*. Río Piedras: Editorial Edil, 1971.

Penco, Wilfredo. *José Enrique Rodó*. Montevideo: Arca, 1978.

Perus, Françoise. *Historia y crítica literaria: el realismo social y la crisis de la dominación oligárquica*. Havana: Casa de las Américas, 1982.

Pick, Daniel. *Faces of Degeneration. A European Disorder, c.1848-c.1918.* Cambridge: Cambridge University Press, 1993.

del Pino, C. Castilla. "Para una patografía de Ángel Ganivet." *Ínsula,* nos. 228-229 (1965).

Platt, Tristan. "The Andean Experience of Bolivian Liberalism, 1825-1900: Roots of Rebellion in 19th-Century Chayanta (Potosí)." *Resistance, Rebellion and Consciousness in the Andean Peasant World, 19th to 20th Centuries.* Ed. Steve J. Stern. Madison: The University of Wisconcin Press, 1987.

Pratt, Mary Louise. *Imperial Eyes: Studies in Travel Writing and Transculturation.* London and New York: Routledge, 1992.

Rama, Ángel. *Rubén Darío y el modernismo.* Caracas: Universidad Central de Venezuela, 1970.

Rama, Carlos. *Historia de las relaciones culturales entre España y la América Latina.* Mexico: Fondo de Cultura Económica, 1982.

Ramos, Julio. *Desencuentros de la modernidad en América Latina. Literatura y política en el siglo XIX.* Mexico: Fondo de Cultura Económica, 1989.

Ramsden, H. *Angel Ganivet's Idearium español: A Critical Study.* Manchester: University of Manchester Press, 1967.

———. *The 1898 Movement in Spain. Towards a Reinterpretation with Special Reference to En torno al casticismo and Idearium español.* Manchester: Manchester University Press, 1974.

Rangel, Carlos. *Del Buen Salvaje al Buen Revolucionario.* Buenos Aires: Monte Ávila Editores, C.A., 1976.

Real de Azúa, Carlos. Prologue. *Ariel.* By José Enrique Rodó. (1900) Edition by Ángel Rama. Caracas: Biblioteca Ayacucho, 1976.

Ribot, Théodule. *Heredity: A Psychological Study of its Phenomena, Laws and Causes.* New York: D. Appleton and Co., 1875.

Roca, José Luis, *Epistolario de Alcides Arguedas: la generación de la amargura.* La Paz: Última Hora, 1979.

Rodó, José Enrique. *Ariel. Liberalismo y Jacobinismo.* Mexico: Editorial Porrúa, S.A., 1977. 1-59.

———. *La América Nuestra.* Compilation and Prologue by Arturo Ardao. Havana: Casa de las Américas, 1977.

———. *Rubén Darío,* in *Ariel. Liberalismo y Jacobinismo.* Mexico: Editorial Porrúa, S.A., 1977. 137-170.

Rodríguez-Luis, Julio. *Hermenéutica y praxis del indigenismo.* Mexico: Fondo de Cultura Económica, 1989.

Romero Baró, José María. *El positivismo y su valoración en América.* Barcelona: Promociones Publicaciones Universitarias, 1989.

Schopenhauer. *On the Will in Nature.* Trans. E.F.J. Payne. Ed. David E. Cartwright. New York: Berg, 1992.

———. *The World as Will and Representation.* Trans. E.F.J. Payne. 2 vols. New York: Dover, 1969.

Schorske, Carl E. *Fin-De-Siècle Vienna. Politics and Culture.* New York: Vintage Books, 1981.

Sedgwick, Eve Kosofsky. *Between Men: English Literature and Male Homosexual Desire.* New York: Columbia University Press, 1985.

———. *Epistemology of the Closet.* Berkeley and Los Angeles: University of California press, 1990.

Senabre, Ricardo. "Ganivet y el diagnóstico de la abulia." In *Studia hispanica in honorem R. Lapesa,* vol. 2, Madrid: Gredos, 1974. 595-99.

Shakespeare, William. *The Tempest. The Complete Works of William Shakespeare.* New York: Avenal Books, 1975.

Siles Guevara, Juan. *Las cien obras capitales de la literatura boliviana*. La Paz: Editorial "Los Amigos del Libro," 1975.

Silk, M.S. and Stern, J.P. *Nietzsche on Tragedy*. Cambridge: Cambridge University Press, 1984.

Smith, Paul Julian. *The Body Hispanic: Gender and Sexuality in Spanish and Spanish American Literature* NY: Oxford University Press, 1989.

Sobejano, Gonzalo. *Nietzsche en España*. Madrid: Gredos, 1967.

Sommer, Doris. "Irresistible Romance: the Foundational Fictions of Latin America." *Nation and Narration*. Ed. Homi K. Bhabha. New York: Routledge, 1990. 71-98.

Spackman, Barbara. *Decadent Genealogies. The Rhetoric of Sickness from Baudelaire to D'Annunzio*. Ithaca: Cornell University Press, 1989.

Stabb, Martin S. *In Quest of Identity. Patterns in the Spanish American Essay of Ideas, 1890-1960*. Chapel Hill: University of North Carolina Press, 1967.

Stekel, Wilhelm. *Compulsion and Doubt*. trans. Emil A. Gutheil, M.D. 2 vols. New York: Liverwright Publishing Corp., 1949.

———. *The Homosexual Neurosis*. Trans. James Van Treslaar, M.D. New York: Emerson Books, Inc., 1945.

Stepan, Nancy. "Biology and Degeneration: Races and Proper Places." *Degeneration: The Dark Side of Progress*. Eds. J. Edward Chamberlin and Sander L. Gilman. New York: Columbia University Press, 1985.

Terán, Óscar. *Positivismo y nación en la Argentina*. Buenos Aires: Puntosur, 1987.

Theweleit, Klaus. *Male Fantasies. Volume 2 Male Bodies: Psychoanalyzing the White Terror*. Trans. Erica Carter and Chris Turner. Minneapolis: University of Minnesota Press, 1989.

Tzitsikas, Helene. *El sentimiento ecológico en la generación del 98*. Barcelona: Borrás Ediciones, 1977.

Ugarte, Manuel. *Enfermedades sociales*. Barcelona: Casa Editorial Sopena, 1907.

Unamuno, Miguel de. *En torno al casticismo*. Madrid: Colección Austral, 1977 ed.

Viñas, David. "De los gentlemen-escritores a la profesionalización de la literatura." *Literatura argentina y realidad política*. Buenos Aires: Centro Editor de América Latina, 1982.

Weininger, Otto. *Sex and Character*. 1903. New York: AMS Press Inc., 1975. Reprint of 1906 ed.

Williams, Raymond. "Social Darwinism" in *Problems in Materialism and Culture*. London: Verso, 1980. 86-102.

Zuleta, Ignacio. *La polémica modernista: el modernismo de mar a mar (1898-1907)*. Bogota: Publicaciones del Instituto Caro y Cuervo, 1988.

NORTH CAROLINA STUDIES IN THE ROMANCE LANGUAGES AND LITERATURES

I.S.B.N. Prefix 0-8078-

Recent Titles

DISCOVERING THE COMIC IN "DON QUIXOTE", by Laura J. Gorfkle. 1993. (No. 243). -9247-5.

THE ARCHITECTURE OF IMAGERY IN ALBERTO MORAVIA'S FICTION, by Janice M. Kozma. 1993. (No. 244). -9248-3.

THE "LIBRO DE ALEXANDRE". MEDIEVAL EPIC AND SILVER LATIN, by Charles F. Fraker. 1993. (No. 245). -9249-1.

THE ROMANTIC IMAGINATION IN THE WORKS OF GUSTAVO ADOLFO BÉCQUER, by B. Brant Bynum. 1993. (No. 246). -9250-5.

MYSTIFICATION ET CRÉATIVITÉ DANS L'OEUVRE ROMANESQUE DE MARGUERITE YOURCENAR, par Beatrice Ness. 1994. (No. 247). -9251-3.

TEXT AS TOPOS IN RELIGIOUS LITERATURE OF THE SPANISH GOLDEN AGE, by M. Louise Salstad. 1995. (No. 248). -9252-1.

CALISTO'S DREAM AND THE CELESTINESQUE TRADITION: A REREADING OF CELESTINA, by Ricardo Castells. 1995. (No. 249). -9253-X.

THE ALLEGORICAL IMPULSE IN THE WORKS OF JULIEN GRACQ: HISTORY AS RHETORICAL ENACTMENT IN LE RIVAGE DES SYRTES AND UN BALCON EN FORÊT, by Carol J. Murphy. 1995. (No. 250). -9254-8.

VOID AND VOICE: QUESTIONING NARRATIVE CONVENTIONS IN ANDRÉ GIDE'S MAJOR FIRST-PERSON NARRATIVES, by Charles O'Keefe. 1996. (No. 251). -9255-6.

EL CÍRCULO Y LA FLECHA: PRINCIPIO Y FIN, TRIUNFO Y FRACASO DEL PERSILES, por Julio Baena. 1996. (No. 252). -9256-4.

EL TIEMPO Y LOS MÁRGENES. EUROPA COMO UTOPÍA Y COMO AMENAZA EN LA LITERATURA ESPAÑOLA, por Jesús Torrecilla. 1996. (No. 253). -9257-2.

THE AESTHETICS OF ARTIFICE: VILLIERS'S L'EVE FUTURE, by Marie Lathers. 1996. (No. 254). -9254-8.

DISLOCATIONS OF DESIRE: GENDER, IDENTITY, AND STRATEGY IN LA REGENTA, by Alison Sinclair. 1998. (No. 255). -9259-9.

THE POETICS OF INCONSTANCY, ETIENNE DURAND AND THE END OF RENAISSANCE VERSE, by Hoyt Rogers. 1998. (No. 256). -9260-2.

RONSARD'S CONTENTIOUS SISTERS: THE PARAGONE BETWEEN POETRY AND PAINTING IN THE WORKS OF PIERRE DE RONSARD, by Roberto E. Campo. 1998. (No. 257). -9261-0.

THE RAVISHMENT OF PERSEPHONE: EPISTOLARY LYRIC IN THE SIÈCLE DES LUMIÈRES, by Julia K. De Pree. 1998. (No. 258). -9262-9.

CONVERTING FICTION: COUNTER REFORMATIONAL CLOSURE IN THE SECULAR LITERATURE OF GOLDEN AGE SPAIN, by David H. Darst. 1998. (No. 259). -9263-7.

GALDÓS'S SEGUNDA MANERA: RHETORICAL STRATEGIES AND AFFECTIVE RESPONSE, by Linda M. Willem. 1998. (No. 260). -9264-5.

A MEDIEVAL PILGRIM'S COMPANION. REASSESSING EL LIBRO DE LOS HUÉSPEDES (ESCORIAL MS. h.I.13), by Thomas D. Spaccarelli. 1998. (No. 261). -9265-3.

'PUEBLOS ENFERMOS': THE DISCOURSE OF ILLNESS IN THE TURN-OF-THE-CENTURY SPANISH AND LATIN AMERICAN ESSAY, by Michael Aronna. 1999. (No. 262). -9266-1.

RESONANT THEMES. LITERATURE, HISTORY, AND THE ARTS IN NINETEENTH- AND TWENTIETH-CENTURY EUROPE. ESSAYS IN HONOR OF VICTOR BROMBERT, by Stirling Haig. 1999. (No. 263). -9267-X.

RAZA, GÉNERO E HIBRIDEZ EN EL LAZARILLO DE CIEGOS CAMINANTES, por Mariselle Meléndez. 1999. (No. 264). -9268-8.

When ordering please cite the ISBN Prefix plus the last four digits for each title.

Send orders to: University of North Carolina Press
P.O. Box 2288
CB# 6215
Chapel Hill, NC 27515-2288
U.S.A.

Made in United States
Orlando, FL
22 March 2026